I0704421

ISBN: 9798670653060

30-DAY

QUICK DIET

For Men

METRIC EDITION

Gail Johnson, M.S.
Ron Hill, Jr.

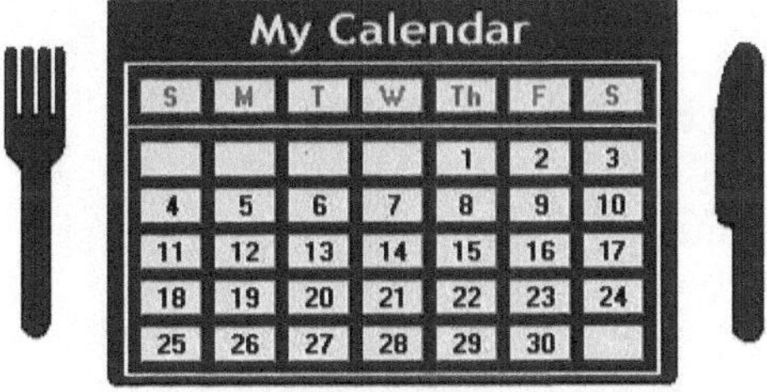

NoPaperPress™

Note: At publication, the off-the-shelf foods used in some of this book were widely available in most supermarkets. But food products come and go. So if there is a frozen entrée or soup selection in this diet that is out of stock, or that's been discontinued, or perhaps you don't like, or that you forgot to pick up while shopping, please substitute another food that has **approximately** the same caloric value and nutritional content.

CONTENTS

Begin with a Medical Exam **(5)**
What's in This eBook?
Which Calorie Level is for You? **(5)**
How Much Weight Will You Lose?
Guidelines for Healthy Eating **(5)**
Exchanging Foods **(7)**
Two Nights Off
Frozen Evening Meals **(8)**
Eating Out
Quick Diet Info **(9)**
Important Notes

1500 kcal DAILY MENUS (11)
Days 1 to 10 **(12)**
Days 11 to 20 **(22)**
Days 21 to 30 **(32)**

1800-kcal DAILY MENUS (43)
Days 1 to 10 **(44)**
Days 11 to 20 **(54)**
Days 21 to 30 **(64)**

RECIPES & DIET TIPS (73)
Day 1 Recipe: Baked Herb-Crusted Cod
Day 2 Recipe: French-Toasted English Muffin **(75)**
Day 3 Recipe: Chicken with Peppers & Onions
Day 4 Recipe: Meat Loaf
Day 5 Recipe: Frozen-Fish Evening Meal
Day 6 Recipe: Grandma's Pizza
Day 7 Recipe: Chicken Evening Meal - Out **(80)**
Day 8 Recipe: Baked Salmon with Salsa
Day 9 Recipe: Veggie Burger
Day 10 Recipe: Wild-Blueberry Pancakes
Day 11 Recipe: Artichoke-Bean Salad
Day 12 Recipe: Fish Evening Meal - Out **(85)**
Day 13 Recipe: Pasta with Marinara Sauce
Day 14 Recipe: Oatena Cereal Mix
Day 15 Recipe: London Broil
Day 16 Recipe: Baked Red Snapper
Day 17 Recipe: Cajun Chicken Salad **(90)**
Day 18 Recipe: Grilled Swordfish
Day 19 Recipe: Chinese Evening Meal - Out
Day 20 Recipe: Quick Pasta alla Puttanesca

Day 21 Recipe: Frozen-Meat Evening Meal
Day 22 Recipe: Shrimp & Spinach Salad **(95)**
Day 23 Recipe: Beans & Greens Salad
Day 24 Recipe: Four Bean Plus Salad
Day 25 Recipe: Hanger Steak
Day 26 Recipe: Grilled Scallops & Polenta
Day 27 Recipe: Fettuccine in Summer Sauce **(100)**
Day 28 Recipe: Frozen Chicken Evening Meal
Day 29 Recipe: Barbequed Shrimp
Day 30 Recipe: Cheeseburger **(103)**

Appendix A Frozen Entrees (104)
Appendix B Frozen Food Safety (109)
Appendix C Soup Selections (110)

NoPaperPress Paperbacks and eBooks (111)

Disclaimer

Begin with a Medical Exam

Everyone should at the very least have a medical assessment, or exam, before starting a weight loss diet. Why? You need to make sure your health will allow you to lower your caloric intake and increase your physical activity. The medical checkup may be as simple as a visit to a physician who is familiar with your medical history, or it may be a thorough physical exam. The physician conducting the medical exam should be made aware of and should approve the specific weight loss diet you're planning.

What's in This eBook?

This eBook actually contains two 30-day diets: a 1800 kcal diet, and for even faster weight loss a 1500 kcal diet. And both diets have a meal plan (menu) for each and every one of the 30 days.

Which Calorie Level is for You?

1500 kcal Quick Diet: Smaller men, older men and inactive men should select the 1500 kcal diet.

1800 kcal Quick Diet: Larger men, younger men and active men should choose the 1800 kcal diet.

How Much Weight Will You Lose?

Weight loss occurs when your food energy intake is less than the total energy you expend. This difference in calories is referred to as your <u>calorie deficit</u>. How much weight you lose depends on the magnitude of your calorie deficit. Simple metabolic calculations make a rough estimate possible. **On the 30-Day Quick Diet, <u>most men lose 7 to 9 kilos</u> –** depending on whether the 1800 or 1500 kcal diet is selected. Smaller men, older men and less active men will lose a bit less and larger men, younger men and more active men often lose much more. Exactly how much weight you will lose depends on how much you weigh, your age and your activity level. For the full story see *Weight Control - Metric Edition* by Vincent Antonetti, Ph.D.

Guidelines for Healthy Eating

No single food can supply all the nutrients you need in the amounts you need. The most important factors in nutrition are variety, variety, variety! **Variety is the key to a nutritious diet.** As a means of setting strategies for food selection, the U.S. Department of Health and Human Services and the Department of Agriculture issue Dietary Guidelines every five years.

The latest Dietary Guidelines describe a healthy diet as one that:
- Emphasizes fruits, vegetables, whole grains, and fat-free or low-fat milk products.
- Includes fish, poultry, lean meats, beans and nuts.
- Is low in saturated fats, trans fats, cholesterol, salt (sodium) and added sugars.

The guidelines encourage adults to consume a variety of nutrient-dense foods and beverages within their caloric needs. The afore mentioned U.S. government agency recommends how much should be eaten from each of the basic food groups (i.e., from the fruit group, vegetable group, grains group, meat and beans group, milk group, and oils group) – whether you are trying to lose weight or maintain your weight. All this information and more can be found in my eBook *Eat Smart - Metric Edition* published by NoPaperPress.

Even though most adults can get all the vitamins and minerals they need by merely consuming a variety of nutritious foods (from the fruit group, the vegetable group, the grains group, the meat and beans group, the milk group, and the oils group), many physicians recommend a daily multi-vitamin/mineral supplement – just in case you don't eat the way you should.

Large Green Salad: One of the Evening Meals mainstays is a "Large Green Salad." Prepare your "Large Green Salad" in a bowl with a volume of at least 500 mL. First add about 1 cup of either green leaf lettuce, Romaine lettuce or a mesclun mix. Then add, as desired, half cup of green veggies such as broccoli, celery, cucumber, peppers, spinach, or watercress. This vegetable combination will, on average, total about 35 kcal. You will be eating a "Large Green Salad" just about every day at dinnertime. Remember that variety is the key to a nutritious diet. So be sure to vary the ingredients of the salad.
Top your "Large Green Salad" with about <u>20 mL of any light salad dressing</u> available at your local supermarket that contains no more than 2 kcal per mL.
Your "Large Green Salad" with salad dressing will cost you roughly 70 kcal but will be packed with lots of health-giving vitamins, minerals and fiber.

About Bread: First understand that bread, more specifically whole-grain breads, are good sources of complex carbohydrates and dietary fiber, as well as several B vitamins (thiamin, riboflavin, niacin, and foliate), vitamin E, and minerals (iron, magnesium and selenium). In recent years, however, sliced bread loaves have gotten larger, as have the bread slices inside these loaves. Just a few years ago the standard slice of bread contained about 65 to 70 kcal – now most are 100 plus kcal.

   The *30-Day Quick Diet* requires whole-grain bread at 65 to 70 kcal per slice. Quite a few bakers sell thin sliced or "light" sliced bread. The difficult part is finding a whole grain thin sliced or "light" bread (with about 70 kcal per slice). Whatever the brand, make sure the first word in the Ingredients list is "whole." "Pepperidge Farm Small Slice 100% Whole Wheat" is a good choice. It's whole grain, has 70 kcal per slice and tastes good too.

Exchanging Foods

If there is a food listed in the *30-Day Quick Diet* that you don't like, or perhaps that you forgot to pick up while shopping, you probably can exchange or substitute another food in its place – a technique used by dieticians. Exchanging a food listed in a diet for another food with approximately equal caloric value and nutritional content is the foundation of a successful long-term diet. Substitution possibilities are almost endless but have to be done carefully.

   The easiest substitutions are those within the same food group, such as exchanging one vegetable variety for another, or a glass of milk for a cup of yogurt. More sophisticated exchanges cross food groups, for instance replacing 150 grams of chicken breast with 30 grams of peanut butter spread on a piece of whole grain bread. Both foods are complete protein and both contain about 260 kcal.

   Refer to a good calorie table and with some understanding and experience, you can use the table to help you substitute foods called for in the *30-Day Quick Diet* with equal calorie foods from the same food group.

Breakfast: You may substitute any cereal for any other wholesome cereal. For example, if you're not crazy about having Shredded Wheat for breakfast on Day 6, substitute Weetabix, etc. If you don't like the soft-boiled egg called for on Day 9, make yourself a scrambled egg instead. And if Cantaloupe is on the menu but is not in season, replace the cantaloupe with a half cup of orange juice.

Snacks: Again, where yogurt is specified you may substitute an 8-ounce glass of skim milk, but to maintain a nutritionally balanced diet keep this snack a dairy selection. Similarly, when fruit is on the agenda, you may select another type of fruit but do not stray from the fruit group. Nuts and popcorn can be interchanged at will. (Incidentally, you consider buying a hot-air popper. They make great popcorn – which is high in fiber and makes a tasty and nutritious snack.)

Two Nights Off

Everyone deserves a break from the grind of preparing dinner after coming home from work. So the *30-Day Quick Diet* gives you two days off per week! Notice that one night a week the meal plan calls for a frozen dinner and on a second night during the week you're encouraged to eat out. There are, however, some rules and caveats involved and these are covered in the next two sections.

Frozen Dinners

In general, a frozen dinner should not be a meal in itself. Make sure you add a salad, fruit, bread etc. The frozen dinner you choose should come with at least one cup of cooked vegetables. If your frozen dinner doesn't measure up, add your own frozen, fresh or canned vegetables. And look for dinners with no more than 800 mg of sodium. In addition, make sure the dinner you choose has no more than 30 percent of the daily value for total fat. To choose a frozen entrée, go to our extensive tabulation in Appendix A - page 104.

And on the days when a frozen dinner is specified, you will also be given a calorie goal for the frozen dinner. For example, Day 5 calls for frozen fish dinner with a maximum allowable 300 kcal. If you choose a frozen fish dinner that contains less than 300 kcal, you may spend the unused calories any way you wish.

Moreover, on those nights when you just don't have the energy or time to cook, you can always substitute a frozen dinner for the entree listed in the meal plan. For example, Day 1 calls for Herb-Crusted Cod for dinner. The total calorie count for dinner is 525. In place of the cod, any combination of a frozen fish dinner and side dishes (salads, etc) with a total calorie content close to 525 would be an acceptable, albeit not as tasty, alternative.

Eating Out

You may eat out once a week. When you're on a diet, however, eating in a restaurant can be a challenge, because most restaurant portions are huge, and can easily total more than 1000 kcal.

On the *30-Day Quick Diet*, a dinner type (i.e., fish, chicken, etc) and a calorie target is specified. For example Day 7 of the 1500 kcal diet specifies a chicken dinner and allows you 630 kcal.

First, you need to choose a restaurant where you have a fighting chance to achieve your calorie goal. Next, order simple, such as broiled fish with steamed vegetables and brown rice. Tell the waiter you want no sauce, no gravy, nothing added. Then, knowing your calorie objective, and that most fish and chicken are about 200 kcal per 100 grams, most steamed vegetable servings average approximately 40 kcal per 100 grams, rice is about 100 kcal per 100 grams, and a medium baked potato is about 100 kcal, decide how much to eat – and take the remainder home. If fresh fruit is not an option, pass on dessert and have the evening snack specified in the meal plan for that day.

Quick Diet Info

As mentioned previously, there are two diet plans in this eBook:
- 1500 kcal 30-Day Diet starts on page 11.
- 1200 kcal 30-Day Diet starts on page 43.
Both have a detailed meal plan for each of the 30 days. Associated with each day is a "Recipe of the Day" and a "Diet Tip of the Day

The 1200 and 1500 kcal diets adhere to the United States Department of Agriculture recommendation that suggest a balanced diet should have approximately 50 percent of its calories from carbs, about 20 percent from protein sources and 30 percent or less from fat. (Note, the *30-Day Quick Diet* may not be appropriate for individuals with illnesses such as heart disease, diabetes, food allergies, etc. Again, please see your physician before starting this diet – or any diet.)

After you complete the 30th day on the diet, if you still want to lose more weight a good alternative is to repeat the diet by starting over at Day 1.

Important Notes

1) Coffee may be regular or decaf. If desired, skim milk and a sugar substitute may be added to coffee or tea. Soy and almond milk are also acceptable.

2) Fried eggs or scrambled eggs should be cooked in a pan coated with a non-stick cooking spray. Hard-boiled eggs may be substituted for fried, scrambled or soft-boiled eggs.

3) Cereals should be whole grain and unsweetened. At the top of the list are Old-fashioned Oatmeal, Wheatena and Shredded Wheat. Among other reasonably healthy choices are Oatibix, Wheat Chex, Weetabix, some
Kashi cereals and Farina. When blueberries are in season, you may add **blueberries instead of raisins** to your cereal. (Substitution ratio = 2 blueberries per raisin.)

4) Bread may be either plain or toasted whole grain, such as whole grain, whole rye or pumpernickel. Look for whole grain varieties that contain 70 kcal per slice. If desired, bread may be sprayed with a zero-calorie butter substitute. NO BUTTER!

5) When soup is specified, eat only one serving (8 ounces) unless otherwise noted. (Canned soup and microwaveable bowls usually contain about two servings.)

6) Use freely as desired: clear unsweetened coffee, clear unsweetened tea, water, seltzer water and any diet soda, clear soups without fat, bouillon, and seasonings such as mustard, cinnamon, dill, herbs, red and black pepper, curry, vinegar, lemon juice and sections, and dill and sour pickles.

7) Use only lean cuts of meat trimmed of all visible fat. Poultry should be limited to chicken or turkey breasts (white meat only and skinless).

8) When canned tuna or salmon is specified, use only fish packed in water.

9) When the diet calls for turkey bacon, make sure the brand you buy has no more than 35 kcal per slice.

10) An unlimited amount of green salad may be eaten, but the salad dressing should be as specified.

11) Use freely as desired: clear unsweetened coffee, clear unsweetened tea, water, seltzer, any diet soda, clear soups without fat, bouillon, and seasonings such as mustard, cinnamon, dill, herbs, red and black pepper, curry, vinegar, lemon juice and sections, and dill and sour pickles.

12) If it's more convenient, any food item may be moved to any part of the day and combined with any meal or snack.

13) If you cannot find the exact item called for in the diet (because it's out of stock or discontinued), substitute a comparable food (of the same type and close caloric value).

14) Although it's recommended that you follow the diet days as specified, it's fine to occasionally skip a day and/or pick and choose the days you prefer. (Nutritionally, each day stands on its own.)

1500-kcal Daily Menus

Day 1 – 1500 kcal Meal Plan

BREAKFAST	kcal	Totals
Orange juice (120 mL)	50	
Wheat Lakes(30 g) + 120 mL skim milk + ½ banana	190	
Whole-grain toast (1 slice) (See page 7)	65	
Coffee (page 9)	10	315 kcal
SNACK		
Fresh fruit in season (apple, peach, etc)	70	
Coffee or tea	10	80 kcal
MID-DAY MEAL		
Soup (Appendix C - page 110)	110	
Turkey breast (25 g) on 1 slice rye bread (½ sandwich)	105	
Pickle spear	0	
Lettuce & tomato slices	20	
Hot or iced tea	10	245 kcal
SNACK		
Two small cookies (See note at bottom of Day 3)	160	
Skim milk (4 oz)	45	220 Cal
EVENING MEAL		
Baked Herb-Crusted Cod (Day 1 Recipe - page 74)	230	
Spinach (½ cup) steamed with garlic & drizzled with	100	
Asparagus (7 spear cooked & drained)	20	
Baked potato (medium)	100	
Whole-grain bread (1 slice)	65	
Water with lemon section	15	530 kcal
SNACK		
Popcorn Mini Bag*	110	
Coffee or tea	10	120 kcal
* For example Orville Redenbacher's Smart Pop		1510 kcal

Day 2 – 1500 kcal Meal Plan

BREAKFAST	kcal	Totals
Fresh or frozen strawberries (75 g)	25	
French toasted English Muffin (**Day 2 Recipe** - page 75)	270	
Light syrup (15 mL)	30	
Coffee	10	335 kcal
SNACK		
Yogurt (100 g, nonfat, any flavor)	90	
Coffee or tea	10	100 kcal
MID-DAY MEAL		
Salad (90 g tuna, 1 tsp Evoo, onions & celery)	175	
Lettuce & tomato wedges	20	
Rye bread (1 slice)	65	
Fresh fruit in season (apple, plum, etc)	70	
Coffee or tea	10	340 kcal
SNACK		
Handful unsalted mixed nuts	100	
Coffee or tea	10	110 kcal
EVENING MEAL		
Broiled veal chop (120 g lean)	200	
Corn on the cob (1 medium ear)	100	
Broccoli (75 g steamed & drizzled with 5 mL Evoo)	70	
Large green salad with 25 mL low-cal dressing*	70	
Water with lemon wedge	15	455 kcal
* See page 6.		
SNACK		
Crackers or biscuits**	150	
Coffee or tea	10	160 kcal
** Number of crackers / biscuits determined by calorie total.		1500 kcal

Day 3 – 1500 kcal Meal Plan

BREAKFAST	kcal	Totals
Grapefruit (½)	75	
Scrambled egg (Notes - page 9)	80	
Turkey bacon (1 slice)	35	
Whole grain toast (1 slice)	65	
Coffee	10	265 kcal
SNACK		
Yogurt (100 g, nonfat, any flavor)	90	
Coffee or tea	10	100 kcal
MID-DAY MEAL		
Ham (60 g) with mustard on 2 slices rye bread	290	
Small bunch of grapes	65	
Gelatin dessert (unsweetened)	10	
Hot or iced tea	10	375 kcal
SNACK		
Popcorn Mini Bag	110	
Coffee or tea	10	120 kcal
EVENING MEAL		
Chicken w Peppers & Onions (Day 3 Recipe - page 76)	250	
Sautéed red peppers with onions	70	
Green beans - steamed & mashed cauliflower	45	
Large green salad with 25 mL low-cal dressing	70	
Whole-grain bread (1 slice)	65	
Fresh fruit in season (apple, plum, etc)	70	570 kcal
SNACK		
One small cookie*	80	
Coffee or tea	10	90 kcal
* Oatmeal, ginger snap, sugar, etc - check calories!		1520 kcal

Day 4 – 1500 kcal Meal Plan

BREAKFAST	kcal	Totals
Grapefruit (½)	75	
Cheerios (30 g) + ½ cup skim milk + about 15 raisins*	190	
Coffee	10	275 kcal
SNACK		
Fresh fruit in season (apple, peach, etc)	70	
Coffee or tea	10	80 kcal
MID-DAY MEAL		
Subway Sandwich (Ham, Cheese + veggies)*	260	
Canned pineapple (240 mL, no-sugar-added juice)	80	
Water with lemon wedge	10	350 kcal
* On 6" half wheat roll.		
SNACK		
Handful unsalted mixed nuts	100	
Coffee or tea	10	110 kcal
EVENING MEAL		
Meat Loaf (Day 4 Recipe - page 77)	290	
One-half acorn squash (baked w 3 mL maple syrup)	90	
Spinach (75 g steamed & drizzled with 3 mL Evoo)	70	
Romaine lettuce, tomato slices & 15 mL low-cal dressing	45	
Gelatin dessert (unsweetened)	10	
Water with lemon section	15	520 kcal
SNACK		
Two small cookies	160	
Coffee or tea	10	170 kcal
* See page 10 re substituting blueberries for raisins.		1505 kcal

Day 5 – 1500 kcal Meal Plan

BREAKFAST	kcal	Totals
Cantaloupe (½ medium)	50	
Fried egg	80	
Toasted raisin bread (1 slice)	75	
Coffee	10	215 kcal
SNACK		
Yogurt (120 g, nonfat, any flavor)	90	
Coffee or tea	10	100 kcal
MID-DAY MEAL		
Soup (Appendix C - page 110)	140	
Small whole-grain roll	80	
Lettuce & tomato with 15 mL low-cal dressing	45	
Canned pineapple (½ cup, no-sugar-added juice)	40	
Hot or iced tea	10	315 kcal
SNACK		
Popcorn Mini Bag	110	
Coffee or tea	10	120 kcal
EVENING MEAL		
Frozen fish Evening Meal (Day 5 Recipe - page 78)	340	
Large green salad with 25 mL low-cal dressing	70	
Whole-grain bread (1 slice)	65	
Fresh fruit in season (apple, peach, etc)	70	
Water with lemon section	15	560 kcal
SNACK		
Crackers or biscuits	120	
Skim milk (180 mL)	70	190 kcal
* Number of crackers / biscuits determined by calorie total.		1500 kcal

Day 6 – 1500 kcal Meal Plan

BREAKFAST	kcal	Totals
Tomato juice (120 mL)	20	
Shredded Wheat (50 g) + 120 mL milk + ½ banana	265	
Coffee	10	295 kcal
SNACK		
Handful unsalted mixed nuts	100	
Coffee or tea	10	110 kcal
MID-DAY MEAL		
Leftover meat loaf (½ Day 4 serving) with ketchup	155	
Small whole-grain roll	80	
Lettuce	0	
Fresh or frozen berries (75 g)	50	
Hot or iced tea	10	295 kcal
SNACK		
Yogurt (100 g, nonfat, any flavor)	90	
Coffee or tea	10	100 kcal
EVENING MEAL		
Pizza (Day 6 Recipe - page 79)	350	
Large green salad with 25 mL low-cal dressing	70	
Fresh fruit in season (peach, plum, etc)	70	
Glass of red wine (120 mL)	100	
Water with lemon section	15	605 kcal
SNACK		
Crackers or biscuits	90	
Coffee or tea	10	100 kcal
* Number of crackers / biscuits determined by calorie total.		1505 kcal

Day 7 – 1500 kcal Meal Plan

BREAKFAST	kcal	Totals
Cantaloupe (½ medium)	**50**	
Oatmeal (40 g) + 120 mL skim milk + about 15 raisins	**220**	
Coffee	**10**	**280 kcal**
SNACK		
Fresh fruit in season (pear, plum, etc)	**70**	
Coffee or tea	**10**	**80 kcal**
MID-DAY MEAL		
Soup (Appendix C - page 110)	**100**	
Grilled cheese sandwich (2 slices 2% thedcheese)	**230**	
Lettuce and sliced tomato	**20**	
Pickle spear	**0**	
Water	**0**	**350 kcal**
SNACK		
Carrot sticks + ¼ cup low-fat cottage cheese & chives	**60**	
Coffee or tea	**10**	**70 kcal**
EVENING MEAL		
Eat Out – Chicken dinner (Day 7 Recipe - page 80)		
Max allowable calories	**630**	**630 kcal**
	0	
SNACK		
Crackers or biscuits	**90**	
Coffee or tea	**10**	**100 kcal**
		1510 kcal

Day 8 – 1500 kcal Meal Plan

BREAKFAST	kcal	Totals
Cantaloupe (½ medium)	50	
Wheaties (30 g) + 120 mL skim milk + ½ banana	190	
Whole-grain toast (1 slice)	65	
Coffee	10	315 kcal
SNACK		
Fresh fruit in season (apple, peach, etc)	70	
Coffee or tea	10	80 kcal
MID-DAY MEAL		
Soup (Appendix C - page 110)	130	
Turkey (30 g) on 1 slice of rye bread (½ sandwich)	115	
Lettuce & tomato slices	20	
Hot or iced tea	10	275 kcal
SNACK		
Two small cookies	160	
Skim milk (120 mL)	40	200 kcal
EVENING MEAL		
Baked salmon with salsa (Day 8 Recipe - page 81)	215	
Summer squash, zucchini and tomatoes	60	
Brown rice (100 g)	100	
Large green salad with 25 mL low-cal dressing	70	
Fresh fruit in season (apple, plum, etc)	70	
Water with lemon wedge	15	515 kcal
SNACK		
Popcorn Mini Bag	110	
Coffee or tea	10	120 kcal
		1505 kcal

Day 9 – 1500 kcal Meal Plan

BREAKFAST	kcal	Totals
Orange juice (120 mL)	50	
Soft-boiled egg	80	
Whole-grain toast (2 slices)	130	
Coffee	10	270 kcal
SNACK		
Yogurt (120 g, nonfat, any flavor)	90	
Coffee or tea	10	100 kcal
MID-DAY MEAL		
Salad (90 g tuna, 1 tsp Evoo, onions & celery)	175	
Lettuce & tomato wedges + rye bread (1 slice)	85	
Fresh fruit in season – (apple, pear, etc)	70	
Gelatin dessert (unsweetened)	10	
Coffee or tea	10	350 kcal
SNACK		
Handful unsalted mixed nuts	100	
Coffee or tea	10	110 kcal
EVENING MEAL		
Veggie burger (1 patty) (Recipe 9 - page 82)	100	
Low-fat cheddar cheese (1 thin slice)	50	
Seeded hamburger roll + Beets (3 small)	185	
Large green salad with 25 mL low-cal dressing	70	
Fresh fruit in season (apple, peach, etc)	70	
Hot or iced tea	10	485 kcal
SNACK		
Crackers or biscuits	120	
Skim milk (180 mL)	70	190 kcal
		1505 kcal

Day 10 – 1500 kcal Meal Plan

BREAKFAST	kcal	Totals
Orange juice (½ cup)	50	
Wild blueberry pancakes (Day 10 Recipe - page 83)	190	
Turkey bacon (2 slices)	70	
Light syrup (25 mL)	45	
Coffee	10	365 kcal
SNACK		
Yogurt (120 g, nonfat, any flavor)	90	
Coffee or tea	10	100 kcal
MID-DAY MEAL		
Peanut butter (30 g) on 2 slices whole-grain bread	330	
Skim milk (120 mL)	45	
Fresh fruit in season (apple, peach, etc)	70	445 kcal
SNACK		
Popcorn Mini Bag	110	
Coffee or tea	10	120 kcal
EVENING MEAL		
Broiled pork chop (about ½" thick & trimmed of fat)	260	
Green peas (75 g)	55	
Tomato & cucumber salad with 2 Tbsp low-cal dressing	70	
Water	0	385 kcal
SNACK		
Fiber One Chocolate Fudge Brownie*	90	
Coffee or tea	10	100 kcal
* If unavailable an equivalent dessert.		1515 kcal

Day 11 – 1500 kcal Meal Plan

BREAKFAST	kcal	Totals
Fresh sliced orange	75	
Cheerios (30 g) + 120 mL skim milk + about 15 raisins	190	
Whole-grain toast (1 slice)	65	
Coffee	10	340 kcal
SNACK		
Fresh fruit in season (pear, plum, etc)	70	
Coffee or tea	10	80 kcal
MID-DAY MEAL		
Subway Sandwich (Ham, Cheese + veggies)*	260	
Canned pineapple (1 cup, no-sugar-added juice)	80	
Diet soda or water	0	340 kcal
* On 6" half wheat roll.		
SNACK		
Handful unsalted mixed nuts	100	
Coffee or tea	10	110 kcal
EVENING MEAL		
Grilled chicken sausage (2 links - 70 g per link)	180	
Artichoke-bean salad (Day 11 Recipe - page 84)	190	
Green beans - steamed	25	
Whole-grain bread (1 slice)	65	
Water with lemon section	15	475 kcal
SNACK		
Two small cookies	160	
Coffee or tea	10	170 kcal
		1515 kcal

Day 12 – 1500 kcal Meal Plan

BREAKFAST	kcal	Totals
Grapefruit (½)	75	
Scrambled egg	80	
Turkey bacon (2 slices)	70	
Whole-grain toast (1 slice)	65	
Coffee	10	300 kcal
SNACK		
Yogurt (120 g, nonfat, any flavor)	90	
Coffee or tea	10	100 kcal
MID-DAY MEAL		
Soup (Appendix C - page 110)	160	
Tomato slices + ¼ cup chopped fresh basil + 1 tsp Evoo	60	
Whole-grain bread (1 slice)	65	
Hot or iced tea	10	295 kcal
SNACK		
Fresh fruit in season (apple, plum, etc)	70	
Coffee or tea	10	80 kcal
EVENING MEAL		
Eat Out – Fish Evening Meal (Day 12 Recipe - page 95)		
Max allowable calories	595	595 kcal
	0	
SNACK		
Crackers or biscuits	120	
Coffee or tea	10	130 kcal
		1500 kcal

Day 13 – 1500 kcal Meal Plan

BREAKFAST	kcal	Totals
Orange juice (½ cup)	50	
Shredded Wheat (50 g) + 120 mL skim milk + ½ banana	260	
Coffee	10	320 kcal l
SNACK		
Handful unsalted mixed nuts	100	
Coffee or tea	10	110 kcal
MID-DAY MEAL		
Turkey frank (60 g) with mustard & relish	150	
Hot dog bun	130	
Diet soda or water	0	280 kcal
SNACK		
Yogurt (120 g, nonfat, any flavor)	90	
Coffee or tea	10	100 kcal
EVENING MEAL		
Pasta with Marinara sauce (Day 13 Recipe - page 86)	225	
Large green salad with 25 mL low-cal dressing	70	
Fresh fruit in season (apple, plum, etc)	70	
Italian or French bread (1 slice)	80	
Glass of red wine (120 mL)	100	
Water with lemon section	15	560 kcal
SNACK		
Crackers or biscuits	120	
Coffee or tea	10	130 kcal
		1500 kcal

Day 14 – 1500 kcal Meal Plan

BREAKFAST	kcal	Totals
Cantaloupe (½ medium)	50	
Oatena cereal mix (Day 14 Recipe - page 88)	310	
Whole-grain toast (1 slice)	65	
Coffee	10	435 kcal
SNACK		
Fresh fruit in season (peach, plum, etc)	70	
Coffee or tea	10	80 kcal
MID-DAY MEAL		
Grilled Swiss cheese sandwich (60 g low-fat cheese)	310	
Pickle spear	0	
Gelatin dessert (unsweetened)	10	
Hot or iced tea	10	330 kcal
SNACK		
Handful unsalted mixed nuts	100	
Coffee or tea	10	110 kcal
EVENING MEAL		
Frozen chicken Evening Meal (Day 28 Recipe - page 101)	300	
Large green salad with 25 mL low-cal dressing	70	
Water with lemon section	15	385 kcal
SNACK		
Dark chocolate (30 g)	150	
Coffee or tea	10	160 kcal
		1500 kcal

Day 15 – 1500 kcal Meal Plan

BREAKFAST	kcal	Totals
Fresh or frozen strawberries (1 cup)	50	
French toast (made with 2 slices whole-grain bread)	250	
Light syrup (15 mL)	30	
Coffee	10	340 kcal
SNACK		
Yogurt (120 g, nonfat, any flavor)	90	
Coffee or tea	10	100 kcal
MID-DAY MEAL		
Salad (90 g tuna, 1 tsp Evoo, onions & celery)	175	
Lettuce & tomato wedges	20	
Rye bread (1 slice)	65	
Coffee or tea	10	270 kcal
SNACK		
Handful unsalted mixed nuts	100	
Coffee or tea	10	110 kcal
EVENING MEAL		
London broil (Day 15 Recipe - page 88)	320	
Brown rice 100 g)	100	
Broccoli (150 g steamed)	50	
Fresh fruit in season (apple, plum, etc)	70	
Water with lemon section	15	555 kcal
SNACK		
Crackers or biscuits	120	
Coffee or tea	10	130 kcal
		1505 kcal

Day 16 – 1500 kcal Meal Plan

BREAKFAST	kcal	Totals
Orange juice 120 mL)	50	
Wheat Chex (45 g) + 120 mL skim milk + ½ banana	250	
Coffee	10	310 kcal
SNACK		
Fresh fruit in season (peach, plum, etc)	70	
Coffee or tea	10	80 kcal
MID-DAY MEAL		
Subway 6" Sandwich (Ham, Cheese + veggies)	260	
Hot or iced tea	10	270 kcal
SNACK		
Popcorn Mini Bag	110	
Coffee or tea	10	120 kcal
EVENING MEAL		
Baked red snapper (Day 16 Recipe - page 89)	215	
Wild rice mix	160	
Green beans & tomato	75	
Yogurt (120 g, nonfat, any flavor)	90	
Water	0	540 kcal
SNACK		
Two small cookies	160	
Coffee or tea	10	170 kcal
		1490 kcal

Day 17 – 1500 kcal Meal Plan

BREAKFAST	kcal	Totals
Cantaloupe (½ medium)	50	
Fried egg	80	
Turkey bacon (2 slices)	70	
Toasted raisin bread (1 slice)	75	
Coffee	10	285 kcal
SNACK		
Yogurt (120 g, nonfat, any flavor)	90	
Coffee or tea	10	100 kcal
MID-DAY MEAL		
Soup (Appendix C - page 110)	170	
Lettuce & tomato sandwich (Tbsp light mayo)	170	
Gelatin dessert (unsweetened)	10	
Cucumber slices and carrots and celery sticks	15	
Hot or iced tea	10	375 kcal
SNACK		
Handful unsalted mixed nuts	100	
Coffee or tea	10	110 kcal
EVENING MEAL		
Cajun chicken salad (Day 17 Recipe - page 90)	330	
Whole-grain bread (1 slice)	65	
Fresh fruit in season (apple, peach, etc)	70	
Water with lemon section	15	480 kcal
SNACK		
Dark chocolate (30 g)	150	
Coffee or tea	10	160 kcal
		1510 kcal

Day 18 – 1500 kcal Meal Plan

BREAKFAST	kcal	Totals
Grapefruit (½)	75	
Cheerios (30 g) + 120 mL skim milk + about 15 raisins	190	
Coffee	10	275 kcal
SNACK		
Fresh fruit in season (peach, plum, etc)	70	
Coffee or tea	10	80 kcal
MID-DAY MEAL		
Cottage cheese (225 g low fat)	180	
Large green salad with 25 mL low-cal dressing	70	
Small whole-grain roll	80	
Hot or iced tea	10	340 kcal
SNACK		
Handful unsalted mixed nuts	100	
Coffee or tea	10	110 kcal
EVENING MEAL		
Grilled swordfish (Day 18 Recipe - page 91)	250	
Grilled potatoes	100	
Grilled cherry tomatoes	45	
Spinach (75 g) steamed with garlic & drizzled Evoo	50	
Whole-grain bread (1 slice)	65	
Water with lemon section	15	525 kcal
SNACK		
Two small cookies	160	
Coffee or tea	10	170 kcal
		1500 kcal

Day 19 – 1500 kcal Meal Plan

BREAKFAST	kcal	Totals
Grapefruit (½)	75	
Scrambled egg	80	
Whole-grain toast (1 slice)	65	
Coffee	10	230 kcal
SNACK		
Yogurt (120 g, nonfat, any flavor)	90	
Coffee or tea	10	100 kcal
MID-DAY MEAL		
Subway 6" Sandwich (Roast Beef, Cheese + veggies)	245	
Lettuce & tomato slices	20	
Hot or iced tea	10	275 kcal
SNACK		
Fresh fruit in season (apple, plum, etc)	70	
Coffee or tea	10	80 kcal
EVENING MEAL		
Eat Out – Chinese food (Day 19 Recipe - page 92)		
Max allowable calories	640	640 kcal
SNACK		
Crackers or biscuits	120	
Skim milk (120 mL)	45	165 kcal
		1490 kcal

Day 20 – 1500 kcal Meal Plan

BREAKFAST	kcal	Totals
Tomato juice (½ cup)	20	
Shredded Wheat (50 g) + 120 mL skim milk + ½ banana	260	
Coffee	10	290 kcal
SNACK		
Handful unsalted mixed nuts	100	
Coffee or tea	10	110 kcal
MID-DAY MEAL		
Left over Chinese food from Day 19	260	
Gelatin dessert (unsweetened)	10	
Hot or iced tea	10	280 kcal
SNACK		
Yogurt (6 oz, nonfat, any flavor)	90	
Coffee or tea	10	100 kcal
EVENING MEAL		
Spaghetti alla Puttanesca (Day 20 Recipe - page 93)	345	
Large green salad with 25 mL low-cal dressing	70	
Italian or French bread (1 slice)	80	
Glass of red wine (120 mL)	100	
Water	0	595 kcal
SNACK		
Crackers or biscuits	120	
Coffee or tea	10	130 kcal
		1505 kcal

Day 21 – 1500 kcal Meal Plan

BREAKFAST	kcal	Totals
Cantaloupe (½ medium)	50	
Oatmeal (40 g dry) + 120 mL skim milk + about 15 raisins	220	
Coffee	10	280 kcal
SNACK		
Handful unsalted mixed nuts	100	
Coffee or tea	10	110 kcal
MID-DAY MEAL		
Turkey breast (60 g) sandwich	235	
Lettuce, tomato and 15 mL light mayo	35	
Pickle spear	0	
Fresh fruit in season (apple, plum, etc)	70	
Water	0	340 kcal
SNACK		
Yogurt (120 g, nonfat, any flavor)	90	
Coffee or tea	10	100 kcal
EVENING MEAL		
Frozen meat dinner (Day 21 Recipe - page 94)	300	
Large green salad with 25 mL low-cal dressing	70	
Whole-grain bread (1 slice)	65	
Fresh fruit in season (pear, plum, etc)	70	
Water with lemon section	15	520 kcal
SNACK		
Dark chocolate (30 g)	150	
Coffee or tea	10	160 kcal
		1510 kcal

Day 22 – 1500 kcal Meal Plan

BREAKFAST	kcal	Totals
Fresh or frozen strawberries (½ cup)	25	
French toasted English Muffin (**Day 2 Recipe** - page 75)	270	
Light syrup (15 mL)	30	
Coffee	10	335 kcal
SNACK		
Fresh fruit in season (pear, plum, etc)	70	
Coffee or tea	10	80 kcal
MID-DAY MEAL		
Soup (Appendix C - page 110)	120	
BLT sandwich (2 slices turkey bacon, 1 Tbsp light	235	
Pickle spear	0	
Hot or iced tea	10	365 kcal
SNACK		
Two small cookies	160	
Coffee or tea	10	170 kcal
EVENING MEAL		
Shrimp & spinach salad (**Day 22 Recipe** - page 95)	310	
Whole-grain bread (1 slice)	65	
Large green salad with 25 mL low-cal dressing	70	
Water	0	445 kcal
SNACK		
Yogurt (120 g, nonfat, any flavor)	90	90 kcal
		1495 kcal

Day 23 – 1500 kcal Meal Plan

BREAKFAST	kcal	Totals
Cantaloupe (½ medium)	50	
Wheaties (50 g) + 120 mL skim milk + ½ banana	190	
Whole-grain toast (1 slice)	65	
Coffee	10	315 kcal
SNACK		
Yogurt (120 g, nonfat, any flavor)	90	
Coffee or tea	10	100 kcal
MID-DAY MEAL		
Ham (60 g) with mustard on 2 slices rye bread	290	
Pickle spear	0	
Small bunch of grapes	65	
Hot or iced tea	10	365 kcal
SNACK		
Popcorn Mini Bag	110	
Coffee or tea	10	120 kcal
EVENING MEAL		
Beans & greens salad (Day 23 Recipe - page 96)	260	
Whole-grain bread (1 slice)	65	
Baked potato (medium)	100	
Fresh fruit in season (peach, plum, etc)	70	
Water with lemon section	15	510 kcal
SNACK		
Crackers or biscuits	90	
Coffee or tea	10	100 kcal
		1500 kcal

Day 24 – 1500 kcal Meal Plan

BREAKFAST	kcal	Totals
Fresh orange sliced	75	
Soft-boiled egg	80	
Whole-grain toast (2 slices)	130	
Coffee	10	295 kcal
SNACK		
Handful unsalted mixed nuts	100	
Coffee or tea	10	110 kcal
MID-DAY MEAL		
Salad – 90 g salmon, 1 tsp Evoo, onions & celery	200	
Lettuce & tomato wedges	20	
Rye bread (1 slice)	65	
Fresh fruit in season (apple, peach, etc)	70	
Coffee or tea	10	365 kcal
SNACK		
Popcorn Mini Bag	110	
Coffee or tea	10	120 kcal
EVENING MEAL		
Chicken breast – broiled (150 g)	250	
Four bean plus salad (100 g) Day 24 Recipe - page 97	135	
Large green salad with 25 mL low-cal dressing	70	
Yogurt (120 g, nonfat, any flavor)	90	
Water	0	545 kcal
SNACK		
Fresh fruit in season (apple, plum, etc)	70	
Coffee or tea	10	80 kcal
		1515 kcal

Day 25 – 1500 kcal Meal Plan

BREAKFAST	kcal	Totals
Grapefruit (½)	75	
Cheerios (30 g) + 120 mL skim milk + about 15 raisins	190	
Coffee	10	275 kcal
SNACK		
Fresh fruit in season (apple, peach, etc)	70	
Coffee or tea	10	80 kcal
MID-DAY MEAL		
Cottage cheese (225 g low fat)	180	
Large green salad with 25 mL low-cal dressing	70	
Small whole-grain roll	80	
Hot or iced tea	10	340 kcal
SNACK		
Fiber One Chocolate Fudge Brownie	90	
Coffee or tea	10	100 kcal
EVENING MEAL		
Hanger steak (Day 25 Recipe - page 98)	320	
Roasted potatoes (Day 25 Recipe)	120	
Cherry tomatoes (Day 25 Recipe)	20	
Steamed spinach (50 g)	25	
Whole-grain bread (1 slice)	65	
Water	0	550 kcal
SNACK		
Two small cookies	150	
Coffee or tea	10	160 kcal
		1505 kcal

Day 26 – 1500 kcal Meal Plan

BREAKFAST	kcal	Totals
Cantaloupe (½ medium)	50	
Fried egg	80	
Whole-grain toast (2 slices)	130	
Coffee	10	270 kcal
SNACK		
Handful unsalted mixed nuts	100	
Coffee or tea	10	110 kcal
MID-DAY MEAL		
Soup (Appendix C - page 110)	240	
Hard whole-grain roll (medium)	80	
Lettuce & tomato slices	20	
Gelatin dessert (unsweetened)	10	
Hot or iced tea	10	360 kcal
* Enjoy 2 servings.		
SNACK		
Fresh fruit in season (apple, plum, etc)	70	
Coffee or tea	10	80 kcal
EVENING MEAL		
Grilled scallops (Day 26 Recipe - page 99)	210	
Grilled polenta (Day 26 Recipe)	125	
Mushroom-steamed green beans-red onion, etc	55	
Yogurt (120 g, nonfat, any flavor)	90	
Water with lemon section	15	495 kcal
SNACK		
Crackers or biscuits	120	
Skim milk (180 mL)	70	180 kcal
		1495 kcal

Day 27 – 1500 kcal Meal Plan

BREAKFAST	kcal	Totals
Cantaloupe (½ medium)	50	
Oatmeal (40 g dry) + 120 mL skim milk + about 15 raisins	220	
Coffee	10	280 kcal
SNACK		
Fresh fruit in season (apple, plum, etc)	70	
Coffee or tea	10	80 kcal
MID-DAY MEAL		
Two servings (1 cup) left over Day 24 bean salad	270	
Small whole-grain roll	80	
Lettuce & tomato slices	20	
Hot or iced tea	10	380 kcal
SNACK		
Celery sticks + ¼ cup low-fat cottage cheese & chives	60	
Coffee or tea	10	70 kcal
EVENING MEAL		
Fettuccine (Day 27 Recipe - page 100)	290	
Large green salad with 25 mL low-cal dressing	70	
Italian or French bread (1 slice)	80	
Glass of red wine (120 mL)	100	
Water	0	540 kcal
SNACK		
Dark chocolate (30 g)	150	150 kcal
		1500 kcal

Day 28 – 1500 kcal Meal Plan

BREAKFAST	kcal	Totals
Tomato juice (½ cup)	20	
Shredded Wheat (50 g) + 120 mL skim milk + ½ banana	260	
Coffee	10	290 kcal
SNACK		
Handful unsalted mixed nuts	100	
Coffee or tea	10	110 kcal
MID-DAY MEAL		
Roast beef (60 g) sandwich on whole-grain bread	295	
Lettuce	0	
Fresh fruit in season (peach, plum, etc)	70	
Hot or iced tea	10	375 kcal
SNACK		
Yogurt (120 g, nonfat, any flavor)	90	
Coffee or tea	10	100 kcal
EVENING MEAL		
Frozen chicken dinner (Day 28 Recipe - page 101)	300	
Large green salad with 25 mL low-cal dressing	70	
Whole-grain bread (1 slice)	65	
Fresh fruit in season (peach, plum, etc)	70	
Water	0	505 kcal
SNACK		
Crackers or biscuits	120	
Coffee or tea	10	130 kcal
		1510 kcal

Day 29 – 1500 kcal Meal Plan

BREAKFAST	kcal	Totals
Orange juice (½ cup)	50	
Wild blueberry pancakes (Day 10 Recipe - page 83)	190	
Turkey bacon (2 slices) + Light syrup (30 mL)	130	
Coffee	10	380 kcal
SNACK		
Handful unsalted mixed nuts	100	
Coffee or tea	10	110 kcal
MID-DAY MEAL		
Salad (90 g tuna, 5 mL Evoo, onions & celery)	175	
Lettuce & tomato wedges + Rye bread (1 slice)	85	
Fresh fruit in season (pear, peach, etc)	70	
Coffee or tea	10	340 kcal
SNACK		
Fiber One Chocolate Fudge Brownie	90	
Coffee or tea	10	100 kcal
EVENING MEAL		
Barbequed shrimp (Day 29 Recipe - page 102)	160	
Corn on the cob (medium)	90	
Steamed broccoli (150 g)	50	
Gelatin dessert (unsweetened)	10	
Yogurt (120 g, nonfat, any flavor)	90	
Water	15	400 kcal
SNACK		
Two small cookies	160	
Coffee or tea	10	170 kcal
		1500 kcal

Day 30 – 1500 kcal Meal Plan

BREAKFAST	kcal	Totals
Fresh orange sliced	75	
Wheat Chex (45 g) + 120 mL skim milk + ½ banana	250	
Coffee	10	335 kcal
SNACK		
Fresh fruit in season (peach, plum, etc)	70	
Coffee or tea	10	80 kcal
MID-DAY MEAL		
Subway 6" (Turkey Breast, Cheese + veggies)	230	
Canned pineapple (125 g, no-sugar-added juice)	40	
Hot or iced tea	10	280 kcal
SNACK		
Crackers or biscuits	120	
Coffee or tea	10	130 kcal
EVENING MEAL		
Cheeseburger (Day 30 Recipe - page 103)	320	
Low-fat cheese (1 thin slice)	50	
Lettuce and sliced tomato + Whole-grain hard roll	160	
Steamed green beans	25	
Pickle spear	0	
Water	0	555 kcal
SNACK		
Popcorn Mini Bag	110	
Coffee or tea	10	120 kcal
		1500 kcal

1800-kcal Daily Menus

Day 1 – 1800 kcal Meal Plan

BREAKFAST	kcal	Totals
Orange juice (120 mL)	50	
Wheaties (30 g) + 120 mL skim milk + ½ banana	190	
Whole wheat toast (2 slices)		
Coffee (See Notes page 9)	10	250 kcal l
SNACK		
Fresh fruit in season (apple, peach, etc)	70	
Coffee or tea	10	80 kcal
Mid-Day Meal		
Soup (Appendix C - page 110)	110	
Turkey breast (85 g) on 2 slices rye bread	260	
Lettuce & tomato slices with 30 mL low-cal dressing	70	
Coffee or tea	10	450 kcal
SNACK		
Two small cookies*	160	
Coffee or tea	10	170 kcal
EVENING MEAL		
Baked Herb-Crusted Cod (Day 1 Recipe - page 74)	230	
Spinach (75 g) steamed with garlic & drizzled Evoo	100	
Asparagus (7 spears cooked & drained)	20	
Baked potato (medium)	100	
Large salad with 20 mL low-cal dressing	70	
Whole grain bread (1 slice) (See page 9)	65	
Water with lemon wedge	15	600 kcal
SNACK		
Sorbet (any flavor) 120 mL	120	
Coffee or tea	10	130 kcal
* Oatmeal, ginger snap, sugar, etc - check calories!		1810 kcal

Day 2 – 1800 kcal Meal Plan

BREAKFAST	kcal	Totals
Fresh or frozen strawberries (75 g)	25	
French toasted English Muffin (Day 2 Recipe - page 75)	270	
Light syrup (15 mL)	30	
Coffee	10	335 kcal
SNACK		
Yogurt (120 g, nonfat, any flavor)	90	
Coffee or tea	10	100 kcal
MID-DAY MEAL		
Salad (90 g tuna, 5 mL Evoo, onions & celery)	175	
Lettuce & tomato wedges	20	
Bread (1 slice)	70	
Fresh fruit in season (apple, peach, etc)	70	
Hot or iced tea	10	345 kcal
SNACK		
Handful unsalted mixed nuts	100	
Coffee or tea	10	110 kcal
EVENING MEAL		
Broiled veal chop (180 g lean)	300	
Corn on the cob (1 medium ear)	100	
Broccoli (75 g steamed) drizzled with 5 mL Evoo	95	
Large green salad with 25 mL low-cal dressing*	70	
Non-fat milk (240 mL)	90	
Water	0	395 kcal
* See page 6.		
SNACK		
Crackers or biscuits**	120	
Coffee or tea	10	130 kcal
** Number of crackers / biscuits determined by calorie total.		1810 kcal

Day 3 – 1800 kcal Meal Plan

BREAKFAST	kcal	Totals
Grapefruit (½)	75	
Scrambled egg (2 eggs) (Notes - page 9)	160	
Bacon (2 slices)	90	
Whole wheat toast (2 slices)	130	
Coffee	10	465 kcal
SNACK		
Yogurt (120 g, nonfat, any flavor)	90	
Coffee or tea	10	100 kcal
MID-DAY MEAL		
Ham sandwich (90 g ham & 2 slices rye bread)	370	
Lettuce & tomato slices	20	
Small bunch of grapes	65	
Diet soda or water	0	465 kcal
SNACK		
Fresh fruit in season (apple, peach, etc)	70	
Coffee or tea	10	80 kcal
EVENING MEAL		
Chicken w Peppers & Onions (Day 3 Recipe - page 76)	250	
Sautéed red peppers with onions	70	
Green beans (steamed) & mashed cauliflower	55	
Large green salad with 25 mL low-cal dressing	70	
Whole-grain bread (1 slice)	65	
Non-fat milk (240 mL)	90	600 kcal
SNACK		
Crackers or biscuits	120	
Coffee or tea	10	130 kcal
		1820 kcal

Day 4 – 1800 kcal Meal Plan

BREAKFAST	kcal	Totals
Grapefruit (½)	75	
Cheerios (30 g) + 120 mL milk + about 15 raisins*	190	
Whole-grain toast (1 slice)	65	
Coffee	10	340 kcal
SNACK		
Fresh fruit in season (apple, peach, etc)	70	
Coffee or tea	10	80 kcal
MID-DAY MEAL		
Subway 6" Sandwich (Roast Beef, Cheese + veggies)*	245	
Large tossed salad with 25 mL low-cal dressing	70	
Hot or iced tea	10	325 kcal
* On 6" half wheat roll.		
SNACK		
Handful of unsalted mixed nuts	100	
Coffee or tea	10	110 kcal
EVENING MEAL		
Meat Loaf (1 ½ servings Day 4 Recipe - page 77)	435	
One-half acorn squash (baked w 5 mL maple syrup)	90	
Spinach 75 g steamed & drizzled with 5 mL Evoo)	95	
Romaine lettuce, tomato slices & 15 mL low-cal dressing	45	
Whole-grain bread (1 slice)	65	
Water with lemon wedge	15	745 kcal
SNACK		
Crackers or biscuits	180	
Coffee or tea	10	190 kcal
* See page 10 re substituting blueberries for raisins.		1790 kcal

Day 5 – 1800 kcal Meal Plan

BREAKFAST	kcal	Totals
Cantaloupe (½ medium)	50	
Fried eggs (2 eggs)	160	
Bacon (2 slices)	90	
Toasted raisin bread (2 slices)	150	
Coffee	10	460 kcal
SNACK		
Yogurt (120 g, nonfat, any flavor)	90	
Coffee or tea	10	100 kcal
MID-DAY MEAL		
Soup (Appendix C - page 110)	140	
Small whole-grain roll	80	
Lettuce & sliced tomato w 15 mL low-cal dressing	45	
Canned pineapple (120 mL, no-sugar-added juice)	40	
Hot or iced tea	10	315 kcal
SNACK		
Dark chocolate (30 g)	150	
Coffee or tea	10	160 kcal
EVENING MEAL		
Frozen fish dinner (Day 5 Recipe - page 78)	340	
Large green salad with 25 mL low-cal dressing	70	
Steamed cauliflower (120 g)	25	
Whole-grain bread (1 slice)	65	
Milk - nonfat 240 mL	90	
Fresh fruit in season (apple, peach, etc)	70	660 kcal
SNACK		
Popcorn Mini Bag*	110	
Coffee or tea	10	120 kcal
* For example Orville Redenbacher's Smart Pop		1510 kcal

Day 6 – 1800 kcal Meal Plan

BREAKFAST	kcal	Totals
Tomato juice (½ cup)	20	
Shredded Wheat (50 g) + 120 mL skim milk + ½ banana	265	
Whole-grain toast (2 slices)	130	
Coffee	10	425 kcal
SNACK		
Handful unsalted mixed nuts	100	
Coffee or tea	10	110 kcal
MID-DAY MEAL		
Leftover meat loaf (Day 4 serving size) with ketchup	290	
Small whole-grain roll	80	
Lettuce	0	
Fresh or frozen berries (75 g)	50	
Hot or iced tea	10	430 kcal
SNACK		
Yogurt (6 oz, nonfat, any flavor)	90	
Coffee or tea	10	100 kcal
EVENING MEAL		
Pizza (Day 6 Recipe - page 79)	350	
Large green salad with 25 mL low-cal dressing	70	
Fresh fruit in season (pear, plum, etc)	70	
Glass of red wine (120 mL)	100	
Water with lemon wedge	15	605 kcal
SNACK		
Crackers or biscuits	120	
Coffee or tea	10	130 kcal
		1800 kcal

Day 7 – 1800 kcal Meal Plan

BREAKFAST	kcal	Totals
Cantaloupe (½ medium)	**50**	
Oatmeal (40 g dry) + 120 mL skim milk + about 15 raisins	**220**	
Whole-wheat toast (2 slices)	**130**	
Coffee	**10**	**410 kcal**
SNACK		
Fresh fruit in season (pear, plum, etc)	**70**	
Coffee or tea	**10**	**80 kcal**
MID-DAY MEAL		
Soup (Appendix C - page 110)*	**90**	
Grilled cheese sandwich (2 slices 2% cheese)	**230**	
Lettuce and sliced tomato	**20**	
Pickle spear	**0**	
Hot or iced tea	**10**	**350 kcal**
SNACK		
Popcorn Mini Bag	**110**	
Coffee or tea	**10**	**120 kcal**
EVENING MEAL		
Eat Out – Chicken dinner (Day 7 Recipe - page 80)		
Max allowable calories	**630**	**630 kcal**
SNACK		
Crackers or biscuits	**120**	
Milk - nonfat (240 mL)	**90**	**210 kcal**
		1800 kcal

Day 8 – 1800 kcal Meal Plan

BREAKFAST	kcal	Totals
Cantaloupe (½ medium)	50	
Wheaties (30 g) + 120 mL skim milk + ½ banana	190	
Whole-wheat toast (2 slices)	130	
Coffee	10	380 kcal
SNACK		
Fresh fruit in season (pear, plum, etc)	70	
Coffee or tea	10	80 kcal
MID-DAY MEAL		
Soup (Appendix C - page 110)	140	
Turkey (60 g) on 2 slices of rye bread	230	
Lettuce & tomato slices	20	
Milk - nonfat (240 mL)	90	480 kcal
SNACK		
Two small cookies	160	
Coffee or tea	10	170 kcal
EVENING MEAL		
Baked salmon with salsa (Day 8 Recipe - page 81)	215	
Summer squash, zucchini and tomatoes	60	
Brown rice (150 g)	150	
Large green salad with 25 mL low-cal dressing	70	
Fresh fruit in season (apple, plum, etc)	70	
Water with lemon wedge	15	580 kcal
SNACK		
Popcorn Mini Bag*	110	
Coffee or tea	10	120 kcal
* For example Orville Redenbacher's Smart Pop		1810 kcal

Day 9 – 1800 kcal Meal Plan

BREAKFAST	kcal	Totals
Orange juice (½ cup)	50	
Soft-boiled egg	80	
Bacon (2 slices)	90	
Whole-grain toast (2 slices)	130	
Coffee	10	360 kcal
SNACK		
Yogurt (120 g, nonfat, any flavor)	90	
Coffee or tea	10	100 kcal
MID-DAY MEAL		
Salad (150 g tuna, 5 mL Evoo, onions & celery)	265	
Lettuce & tomato wedges	20	
Rye bread (1 slice)	65	
Fresh fruit in season (pear, peach, etc)	70	
Hot or iced tea	10	430 kcal
SNACK		
Handful unsalted mixed nuts	100	
Coffee or tea	10	110 kcal
EVENING MEAL		
Veggie burger – (1 patty) (Day 9 Recipe - page 82)	100	
Low-fat cheddar cheese (2 thin slices)	100	
Seeded hamburger roll + Beets (3 small)	185	
Large green salad with 25 mL low-cal dressing	70	
Fresh fruit in season (apple, peach, etc)	70	
Nonfat milk (240 mL)	90	615 kcal
SNACK		
Sorbet - any flavor (180 mL)	180	
Coffee or tea	10	190 kcal
		1805 kcal

Day 10 – 1800 kcal Meal Plan

BREAKFAST	kcal	Totals
Orange juice (½ cup)	50	
Wild blueberry pancakes (Day 10 Recipe - page 83)	190	
Bacon (2 slices)	90	
Light syrup (15 mL)	30	
Coffee	10	370 kcal
SNACK		
Yogurt (120 g, nonfat, any flavor)	90	
Coffee or tea	10	100 kcal
MID-DAY MEAL		
Peanut butter (30 g) on 2 slices of whole-grain bread	330	
Skim milk (240 mL)	90	
Fresh fruit in season (apple, plum, etc)	70	490 kcal
SNACK		
Large handful unsalted mixed nuts	150	
Coffee or tea	10	160 kcal
EVENING MEAL		
Soup (Appendix C - page 110)	100	
Broiled pork chop (about ½" thick & trimmed of fat)	260	
Green peas (75 g)	55	
Tomato & cucumber salad 30 mL low-cal dressing	70	
Whole-grain bread (1 slice)	65	
Water with lemon section	15	565 kcal
SNACK		
Popcorn Mini Bag	110	
Coffee or tea	10	120 kcal
		1805 kcal

Day 11 – 1800 kcal Meal Plan

BREAKFAST	kcal	Totals
Fresh sliced orange	75	
Cheerios (30 g) + 120 mL skim milk + about 15 raisins	190	
Whole-wheat toast (2 slices)	130	
Coffee	10	405 kcal
SNACK		
Fresh fruit in season (apple, plum, etc)	70	
Coffee or tea	10	80 kcal
MID-DAY MEAL		
Subway 6" Sandwich (Ham, Cheese + veggies)*	260	
Large tossed salad with 25 mL low-cal dressing	70	
Hot or iced tea	10	340 kcal
SNACK		
Large handful unsalted mixed nuts	150	
Coffee or tea	10	160 kcal
EVENING MEAL		
Grilled chicken sausage (3 links about 70 g per link)	270	
Artichoke-bean salad (Day 11 Recipe - page 84)	190	
Green beans - steamed	25	
Whole-wheat bread (1 slice)	65	
Yogurt (120 g, nonfat, any flavor)	90	
Water with lemon wedge	15	655 kcal
SNACK		
Two small cookies	160	
Coffee or tea	10	170 kcal
		1810 kcal

Day 12 – 1800 kcal Meal Plan

BREAKFAST	kcal	Totals
Grapefruit (½)	75	
Scrambled eggs (2)	80	
Bacon (2 slices)	90	
Whole-grain toast (2 slices)	130	
Coffee	10	465 kcal
SNACK		
Yogurt (120 g, nonfat, any flavor)	90	
Coffee or tea	10	100 kcal
MID-DAY MEAL		
Soup (Appendix C - page 110)	150	
Ham (60 g) on one slice rye bread	225	
Tomato slices, chopped fresh basil + 5 mL Evoo	60	
Hot or iced tea	10	255 kcal
SNACK		
Fresh fruit in season (apple, plum, etc)	70	
Coffee or tea	10	80 kcal
EVENING MEAL		
Eat Out – Fish dinner (Day 12 Recipe - page 85)		
Max allowable calories	595	595 kcal
SNACK		
Crackers or biscuits	90	
Coffee or tea	10	100 kcal
		1795 kcal

Day 13 – 1800 kcal Meal Plan

BREAKFAST	kcal	Totals
Orange juice (120 mL)	50	
Shredded Wheat (50 g) + 120 mL skim milk + ½ banana	260	
Whole-grain toast (2 slices)	130	
Coffee	10	450 kcal
SNACK		
Handful unsalted mixed nuts	100	
Coffee or tea	10	110 kcal
MID-DAY MEAL		
Bologna (60 g) with mustard & relish	150	
Rye bread (2 slices)	130	
Yogurt 120 g, nonfat, & 75 g fresh or frozen berries	140	
Hot or iced tea	10	430 kcal
SNACK		
Crackers or biscuits	120	
Coffee or tea	10	100 kcal
EVENING MEAL		
Pasta with Marinara sauce (Day 13 Recipe - page 86)	225	
Large green salad with 25 mL low-cal dressing	70	
Fresh fruit in season (pear, plum, etc)	70	
Italian or French bread (1 slice)	80	
Glass red wine (120 mL)	100	
Water with lemon section	15	560 kcal
SNACK		
Popcorn Mini Bag	110	
Coffee or tea	10	120 kcal
		1790 kcal

Day 14 – 1800 kcal Meal Plan

BREAKFAST	kcal	Totals
Cantaloupe (½ medium)	50	
Oatena cereal mix (Day 14 Recipe - page 88)	310	
Coffee	10	370 kcal
SNACK		
Handful unsalted mixed nuts	100	
Coffee or tea	10	110 kcal
MID-DAY MEAL		
Grilled Swiss cheese sandwich (60 g low-fat cheese)	310	
Bacon (2 slices)	90	
Hot or iced tea	10	410 kcal
SNACK		
Yogurt (120 g, nonfat, any flavor)	90	
Coffee or tea	10	100 kcal
EVENING MEAL		
Frozen chicken entrée (Appendix A - page 104)	300	
Large green salad with 25 mL low-cal dressing	70	
Fresh fruit in season (pear, plum, etc)	70	
Dark chocolate (30 g)	150	
Water with lemon wedge	15	605 kcal
SNACK		
Crackers or biscuits	150	
Coffee or tea	10	160 kcal
		1780 kcal

Day 15 – 1800 kcal Meal Plan

BREAKFAST	kcal	Totals
Fresh or frozen strawberries (1 cup)	50	
French toast (made with 3 slices whole-grain bread)	375	
Light syrup (30 mL)	60	
Coffee	10	495 kcal
SNACK		
Yogurt (120 g, nonfat, any flavor)	90	
Coffee or tea	10	100 kcal
MID-DAY MEAL		
Salad (150 g tuna, 5 mL Evoo, onions & celery)	265	
Lettuce & tomato wedges	20	
Rye bread (1 slice)	65	
Coffee or tea	10	360 kcal
SNACK		
Handful unsalted mixed nuts	100	
Coffee or tea	10	110 kcal
EVENING MEAL		
London broil (Day 15 Recipe - page 88)	320	
Brown rice (100 g)	100	
Broccoli (150 g steamed)	50	
Fresh fruit in season (pear, plum, etc)	70	
Water	0	540 kcal
SNACK		
Sorbet - any flavor (200 mL)	200	
Coffee or tea	10	210 kcal
		1200 kcal

Day 16 – 1800 kcal Meal Plan

BREAKFAST	kcal	Totals
Orange juice (120 mL)	50	
Wheat Chex (30 g) + 120 mL skim milk + ½ banana	250	
Whole-wheat toast (2 slices)	130	
Coffee	10	440 kcal
SNACK		
Yogurt (120 g, nonfat, any flavor)	90	
Coffee or tea	10	100 kcal
MID-DAY MEAL		
Subway 6" Sandwich (Roast Beef, Cheese + veggies)	245	
Lettuce & tomato slices	20	
Hot or iced tea	10	275 kcal
SNACK		
Two small cookies	160	
Milk Nonfat (240 mL)	90	250 kcal
EVENING MEAL		
Baked red snapper (Day 16 Recipe - page 89)	215	
Wild rice mix - see page 89	160	
Green beans & tomato	75	
Fresh fruit in season (pear, plum, etc)	70	
Water with lemon section	15	600 kcal
SNACK		
Popcorn Mini Bag	110	
Coffee or tea	10	120 kcal
		1785 kcal

Day 17 – 1800 kcal Meal Plan

BREAKFAST	kcal	Totals
Cantaloupe (½ medium)	50	
Fried eggs (2)	160	
Bacon (2 slices)	90	
Toasted raisin bread (2 slices)	150	
Coffee	10	460 kcal
SNACK		
Yogurt (120 g, nonfat, any flavor)	90	
Coffee or tea	10	100 kcal
MID-DAY MEAL		
Soup (Appendix C - page 110)	150	
Lettuce & tomato sandwich with 15 mL light mayo	170	
Cucumber slices and carrot & celery sticks	25	
Hot or iced tea	10	355 kcal
SNACK		
Handful unsalted mixed nuts	100	
Coffee or tea	10	110 kcal
EVENING MEAL		
Cajun chicken salad (Day 17 Recipe - page 90)	330	
Whole-grain bread (1 slice)	65	
Fresh fruit in season (peach plum, etc)	70	
Milk nonfat (240 mL)	90	
Water	0	555 kcal
SNACK		
Dark chocolate (30 g)	150	
Coffee or tea	10	10 kcal
		1790 kcal

Day 18 – 1800 kcal Meal Plan

BREAKFAST	kcal	Totals
Grapefruit (½)	75	
Cheerios (30 g) + 120 mL skim milk + about 15 raisins	190	
Whole-grain toast (2 slices)	130	
Coffee	10	405 kcal
SNACK		
Yogurt (120 g, nonfat, any flavor)	90	
Coffee or tea	10	100 kcal
MID-DAY MEAL		
Cottage cheese (225 g low fat)	180	
Large green salad with 25 mL low-cal dressing	70	
Small whole-grain roll	80	
Hot or iced tea	10	340 kcal
SNACK		
Handful unsalted mixed nuts	100	
Coffee or tea	10	110 kcal l
EVENING MEAL		
Grilled swordfish (Day 18 Recipe - page 91)	250	
Grilled potatoes (page 91)	100	
Grilled cherry tomatoes	45	
Spinach (75 g) steamed with garlic & drizzled Evoo	50	
Whole-grain bread (1 slice)	65	
Fresh fruit in season (peach plum, etc)	70	
Water with lemon section	15	595 kcal
SNACK		
Two small cookies	160	
Milk nonfat (240 mL)	90	250 kcal
		1800 kcal

Day 19 – 1800 kcal Meal Plan

BREAKFAST	kcal	Totals
Grapefruit (½)	75	
Scrambled eggs (2)	160	
Whole-grain toast (2 slices)	130	
Bacon (1 slice)	45	
Coffee	10	420 kcal
SNACK		
Yogurt (120 g, nonfat, any flavor)	90	
Coffee or tea	10	100 kcal
MID-DAY MEAL		
Soup (Appendix C - page 110)	130	
Turkey (60 g) on 2 slices of rye bread	230	
Lettuce & tomato slices	20	
Milk nonfat (180 mL)	60	440 kcal
SNACK		
Fresh fruit in season (apple, plum, etc)	70	
Coffee or tea	10	80 kcal
EVENING MEAL		
Eat Out – Chinese food (Day 19 Recipe - page 92)		
Max allowable calories	640	640 kcal
SNACK		
Sorbet - any flavor (120 mL)	120	
Coffee or tea	10	130 kcal
		1810 kcal

Day 20 – 1800 kcal Meal Plan

BREAKFAST	kcal	Totals
Grapefruit (½)	75	
Shredded Wheat (50 g) + 120 mL skim milk + ½ banana	260	
Raisin bread toast (2 slices)	150	
Coffee	10	495 kcal
SNACK		
Handful unsalted mixed nuts	100	
Coffee or tea	10	110 kcal
MID-DAY MEAL		
Left over Chinese food from Day 19 (see page 92)	260	
Hot or iced tea	10	270 kcal
SNACK		
Yogurt (120 g, nonfat, any flavor)	90	
Coffee or tea	10	100 kcal
EVENING MEAL		
Spaghetti alla Puttanesca (Day 20 Recipe - page 93)	345	
Large green salad with 25 mL low-cal dressing	70	
Italian or French bread (1 slice)	80	
Glass red wine (120 mL)	100	
Water with lemon section	15	610 kcal
SNACK		
Crackers or biscuits	180	
Coffee or tea	10	190 kcal
		1775 kcal

Day 21 – 1800 kcal Meal Plan

BREAKFAST	kcal	Totals
Cantaloupe (½ medium)	50	
Oatmeal (40 g dry) + 120 mL skim milk + about 15 raisins	220	
Whole-grain toast (2 slices)	130	
Coffee	10	410 kcal
SNACK		
Large handful unsalted mixed nuts	150	
Coffee or tea	10	160 kcal
MID-DAY MEAL		
Turkey breast (90 g) sandwich	285	
Lettuce & tomato with 15 mL light mayo	35	
Pickle spear	0	
Fresh fruit in season (apple, plum, etc)	70	
Water with lemon wedge	15	405 kcal
SNACK		
Yogurt 120 g, nonfat, & 75 g fresh or frozen berries	140	
Coffee or tea	10	150 kcal
EVENING MEAL		
Frozen meat dinner (Day 21 Recipe - page 94)	300	
Large green salad with 25 mL low-cal dressing	70	
Whole-grain bread (1 slice)	65	
Water with lemon section	15	450 kcal
SNACK		
Dark chocolate (30 g)	150	
Milk nonfat (240 mL)	90	240 kcal
		1815 kcal

Day 22 – 1800 kcal Meal Plan

BREAKFAST	kcal	Totals
Fresh or frozen strawberries (75 g)	25	
French toasted English Muffins (2) (Day 2 Recipe - page 75)	360	
Light syrup (1 Tbsp)	30	
Coffee	10	425 kcal
SNACK		
Fresh fruit in season (apple, plum, etc)	70	
Coffee or tea	10	80 kcal
MID-DAY MEAL		
Soup (Appendix C - page 110)	140	
BLT sandwich (2 slices bacon, 15 mL light mayo)	245	
Yogurt (120 g, nonfat, any flavor)	90	
Hot or iced tea	10	485 kcal
SNACK		
Two small cookies	160	
Milk nonfat (240 mL)	90	250 kcal
EVENING MEAL		
Shrimp & spinach salad (Day 22 Recipe page 95)	310	
Whole-grain bread (1 slice)	65	
Large green salad with 25 mL low-cal dressing	70	
Water with lemon wedge	15	445 kcal
SNACK		
Popcorn Mini Bag	110	
Coffee or tea	10	120 kcal
		1805 kcal

Day 23 – 1800 kcal Meal Plan

BREAKFAST	kcal	Totals
Cantaloupe (½ medium)	50	
Wheaties (50 g) + 120 mL skim milk + ½ banana	240	
Whole-grain toast (2 slices)	130	
Coffee	10	430 kcal
SNACK		
Yogurt 120 g, nonfat, & 75 g fresh or frozen berries	140	
Coffee or tea	10	150 kcal
MID-DAY MEAL		
Ham (60 g) with mustard on 2 slices rye bread	290	
Pickle spear	0	
Small bunch of grape	65	
Hot or iced tea	10	365 kcal
SNACK		
Handful unsalted mixed nuts	100	
Coffee or tea	10	110 kcal
EVENING MEAL		
Beans & greens salad (Day 23 Recipe - page 96)	260	
Baked potato (medium)	100	
Whole-grain bread (1 slice)	65	
Fresh fruit in season (apple, peach, etc)	70	
Water	0	495 kcal
SNACK		
Two small cookies	160	
Milk nonfat (240 mL)	90	250 kcal
		1800 kcal

Day 24 – 1800 kcal Meal Plan

BREAKFAST	kcal	Totals
Fresh orange sliced	75	
Soft-boiled eggs (2)	160	
Whole-grain toast (2 slices)	130	
Coffee	10	375 kcal
SNACK		
Yogurt 120 g, nonfat, & 75 g fresh or frozen berries	140	
Coffee or tea	10	150 kcal
MID-DAY MEAL		
Salad – 90 g salmon, 5 mL Evoo, onions & celery	200	
Lettuce & tomato wedges	20	
Rye bread (1 slice)	65	
Fresh fruit in season (apple, plum, etc)	70	
Coffee or tea	10	365 kcal
SNACK		
Handful unsalted mixed nuts	100	100 kcal
EVENING MEAL		
Chicken breast – broiled (180 g)	300	
Four bean plus salad (100 g) (Day 24 Recipe - page 97)	135	
Large green salad with 25 mL low-cal dressing	70	
Whole-grain bread (1 slice)	65	
Glass red wine	100	
Water with lemon wedge	15	685 kcal
SNACK		
Popcorn Mini Bag	110	
Coffee or tea	10	120 kcal
		1795 kcal

Day 25 – 1800 kcal Meal Plan

BREAKFAST	kcal	Totals
Grapefruit (½)	75	
Cheerios (1 cup) + ½ cup skim milk + about 15 raisins	190	
Whole-grain toast (2 slices)	130	
Coffee	10	405 kcal
SNACK		
Fresh fruit in season (apple, plum, etc)	70	
Coffee or tea	10	80 kcal
MID-DAY MEAL		
Subway 6" Sandwich (Ham, Cheese + veggies)	260	
Large green salad with 25 mL low-cal dressing	70	
Hot or iced tea	10	340 kcal
SNACK		
Handful unsalted mixed nuts	100	
Coffee or tea	10	110 kcal
EVENING MEAL		
Hanger steak (Day 25 Recipe - page 98)	320	
Roasted potatoes (Day 25 Recipe)	120	
Cherry tomatoes (Day 25 Recipe)	20	
Steamed spinach (½ cup)	25	
Whole-grain bread (1 slice)	65	
Water with lemon wedge	15	565 kcal
SNACK		
Crackers or biscuits	180	
Milk nonfat (240 mL)	90	270 kcal
		1770 kcal

Day 26 – 1800 kcal Meal Plan

BREAKFAST	kcal	Totals
Cantaloupe (½ medium)	50	
Fried eggs (2)	80	
Bacon (2 slices)	90	
Toasted whole-grain bread (2 slices)	130	
Coffee	10	440 kcal
SNACK		
Yogurt (120 g, nonfat, any flavor)	90	
Coffee or tea	10	100 kcal
MID-DAY MEAL		
Soup (Appendix C - page 110)*	300	
Hard whole-grain roll (medium)	80	
Lettuce & tomato slices	20	
Hot or iced tea	10	410 kcal
* Two servings of 150 kcal soup.		
SNACK		
Popcorn Mini bag	110	
Coffee or tea	10	120 kcal
EVENING MEAL		
Grilled scallops (Day 26 Recipe - page 99)	210	
Grilled polenta (Day 26 Recipe)	125	
Mushroom-steamed green beans-red onion	45	
Grilled asparagus	10	
Fresh fruit in season (apple, plum, etc)	70	
Water with lemon wedge	15	475 kcal
SNACK		
Two small cookies	160	
Milk nonfat (240 mL)	90	250 kcal
		1795 kcal

Day 27 – 1800 kcal Meal Plan

BREAKFAST	kcal	Totals
Cantaloupe (½ medium)	50	
Oatmeal (40 g dry) + 120 mL skim milk + about 15 raisins	220	
Whole-grain toast (2 slices)	130	
Coffee	10	410 kcal
SNACK		
Fresh fruit in season (pear, plum, etc)	70	
Coffee or tea	10	80 kcal
MID-DAY MEAL		
Two servings (1 cup) left over Day 24 bean salad	270	
Small whole-grain roll	80	
Lettuce & tomato slices	20	
Yogurt (120 g, nonfat, any flavor)	90	
Hot or iced tea	10	470 kcal
SNACK		
Handful unsalted mixed nuts	100	
Coffee or tea	10	110 kcal
EVENING MEAL		
Fettuccine (Day 27 Recipe - page 100)	290	
Large green salad with 25 mL low-cal dressing	70	
Italian or French bread (1 slice)	80	
Glass red wine (120 mL)	100	
Water with lemon wedge	15	555 kcal
SNACK		
Dark chocolate (30 g)	150	
Coffee or tea	10	160 kcal
		1785 kcal

Day 28 – 1800 kcal Meal Plan

BREAKFAST	kcal	Totals
Tomato juice (120 mL)	20	
Shredded Wheat (50 g) + 120 mL skim milk + ½ banana	260	
Raisin-bread toast (2 slices)	150	
Coffee	10	440 kcal
SNACK		
Handful unsalted mixed nuts	100	
Coffee or tea	10	110 kcal
MID-DAY MEAL		
Roast beef sandwich (90 g) on whole-grain bread	370	
Lettuce & tomato slices	20	
Fresh fruit in season (peach, plum, etc)	70	
Hot or iced tea	10	470 kcal
SNACK		
Yogurt (120 g, nonfat, any flavor)	90	
Coffee or tea	10	100 kcal
EVENING MEAL		
Frozen chicken dinner (Appendix A - page 104)	300	
Large green salad with 25 mL low-cal dressing	70	
Whole-grain bread (1 slice)	65	
Milk non fat (120 mL)	40	
Water	0	475 kcal
SNACK		
Crackers or biscuits	180	
Coffee or tea	10	190 kcal
		1785 kcal

Day 29 – 1800 kcal Meal Plan

BREAKFAST	kcal	Totals
Orange juice (120 mL)	50	
Wild blueberry pancakes (Day 10 Recipe - page 83)	190	
Bacon (2 slices)	90	
Light syrup (25 mL)	45	
Coffee	10	385 kcal
SNACK		
Yogurt 120 g, nonfat & fresh or frozen berries	140	
Coffee or tea	10	150 kcal
MID-DAY MEAL		
Salad (120 g tuna, 5 mL Evoo, onions & celery)	215	
Lettuce & tomato wedges	20	
Rye bread (1 slice)	65	
Fresh fruit in season (apple, peach, etc)	70	
Coffee or tea	10	380 kcal
SNACK		
Large handful unsalted mixed nuts	150	
Coffee or tea	10	160 kcal
EVENING MEAL		
Barbequed shrimp (Day 29 Recipe - page 102)	160	
Corn on the cob (medium)	90	
Steamed broccoli (1 cup equivalent)	50	
Whole-wheat bread (1 slice)	65	
Water with lemon section	15	380 kcal
SNACK		
Crackers or biscuits	240	
Milk non fat (240 mL)	90	330 kcal
		1785 kcal

Day 30 – 1800 kcal Meal Plan

BREAKFAST	kcal	Totals
Fresh orange sliced	75	
Wheat Chex (45 g) + 120 mL skim milk + ½ banana	250	
Whole-wheat toast (2 slices)	130	
Coffee	10	335 kcal
SNACK		
Fresh fruit in season (apple, peach, etc)	70	
Coffee or tea	10	80 kcal
MID-DAY MEAL		
Soup (Appendix C - page 110)	140	
Small whole-grain roll	80	
Raw zucchini slices, celery & carrot sticks	20	
Canned pineapple (125 g, no-sugar-added juice)	40	
Hot or iced tea	10	290 kcal
SNACK		
Popcorn Mini bag	110	110 kcal
EVENING MEAL		
Cheeseburger (Day 30 Recipe - page 103)	320	
Low-fat cheese (2 thin slices)	100	
Lettuce and sliced tomato	20	
Whole-grain hard roll	140	
Steamed green beans	25	
Large green salad with 25 mL low-cal dressing	70	
Water	0	675 kcal
SNACK		
Crackers or biscuits	240	
Milk non fat (240 mL)	90	330 kcal
		1820 kcal

Recipes & Diet Tips

Day 1 Recipe

Baked Herb-Crusted Cod

4 cod fish fillets (120 to 150 grams each)
2 tablespoons flour
2 tablespoons cornmeal
2 tablespoons minced fresh herbs
2 teaspoons lemon juice (10 mL)

Sprinkle cod with lemon juice. Mix flour, cornmeal and herbs and dust the cod with the cornmeal-herb mixture. Bake in oven at 190 °C for 10 minutes. Add salt and black pepper to taste.

Serves 4. One serving is about 230 kcal (for cod only).

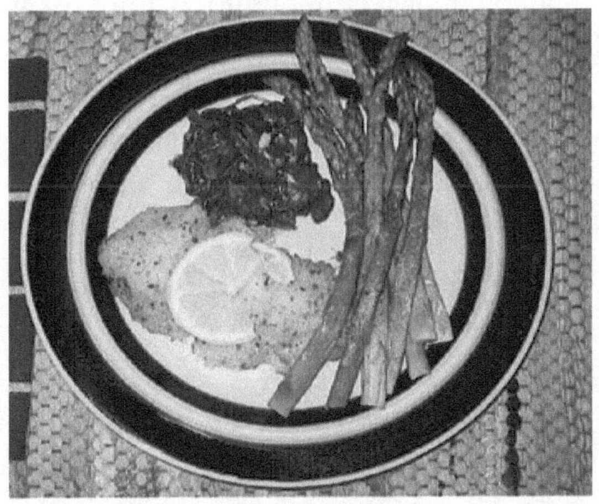

Diet Tip of the Day:. **A reducing diet is best supervised by a physician**. This is especially true when a great deal of weight needs to be lost, or if you have an ailment or a history of medical problems.

Day 2 Recipe
French-Toasted English Muffin

6 whole grain English muffins (light)

4 eggs

2 cups skim milk (480 mL)

2 teaspoons (tsp) vanilla (10 mL)

Dash of cinnamon

In a medium bowl, beat together eggs and skim milk. Add vanilla and cinnamon. Separate English muffins into halves and saturate slices in egg mixture. In a non-stick skillet coated with cooking spray, cook muffins until both sides are golden brown. Dust lightly with confectionary sugar. Serve hot or keep in an oven or warmer at 90 ºC until ready to plate. **Serves 4**. Three English muffin slices (1½ muffins) per serving. Serving is 270 kcal.

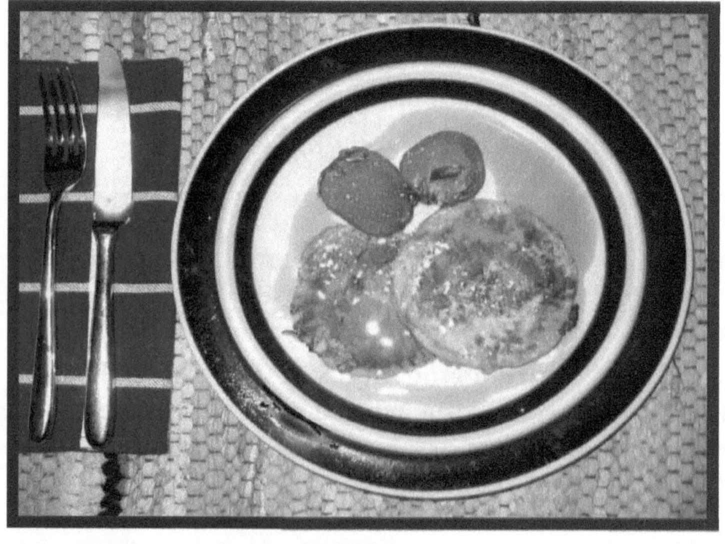

Diet Tip of the Day: "Eat Slowly" This is especially vital when you are trying to lose weight. If you are someone who eats fast, who finishes before everyone else at the table, you are not giving yourself a chance to feel full. While everyone else is still eating, you either sit there and pick, or you have seconds, taking in extra calories you could avoid if you would just slow down.

Day 3 Recipe

Chicken with Peppers & Onions

4 boneless & skinless chicken breasts (~ 150 grams each)
Coat the chicken breasts in a bottled barbeque sauce. Prepare medium-
hot fire on well-oiled gas or charcoal grill . Place breasts on grill, turning
them every 4 minutes, for 10 to 12 minutes, or until done. (To check if
breasts are done, the meat should be moist and white with no sign of pink
when you cut into breast.) Serve hot.
2 medium red peppers
1 medium onion
Place peppers and onions in pan with 2 Tbsp fat-free chicken stock.
Sauté until stock is reduced. Spray pan lightly with non-stick cooking oil
and sauté another 2 minutes. Salt and pepper to taste.
Serves 4. About 250 kcal per serving (for chicken only).

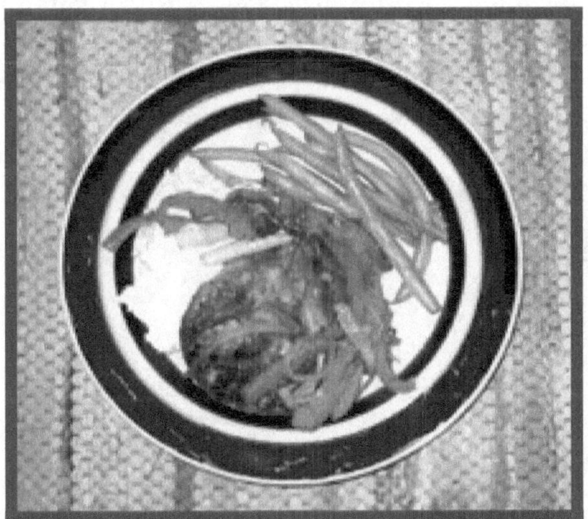

Diet Tip of the Day:. A **reducing diet is best supervised by a
physician**. This is especially true when a great deal of weight needs to be
lost, or if you have an ailment or a history of medical problems.

Day 4 Recipe

Meat Loaf

½ pound (225 grams) ground white meat turkey
½ pound ground beef (about 90% lean)
1 large egg
½ cup (120 mL) skim milk
¼ cup (25 grams) bread crumbs
¼ cup (60 mL) ketchup
¼ cup (30 grams) chopped carrots
¼ cup (30 grams) chopped onion
In a medium bowl, combine all ingredients. Add salt and pepper to taste.
Mix until blended and form into a loaf. Place loaf into oven preheated to
175 ℃. Bake until an instant-read thermometer inserted in the center of
the loaf reads 70 ℃. This should take about one hour.
Shown below is meat loaf, acorn squash baked with 1 tsp (5 mL) maple
syrup and steamed spinach drizzled with extra-virgin olive oil (Evoo).
Serves 5. Each serving of meat loaf is about 290 kcal (for meat loaf only).

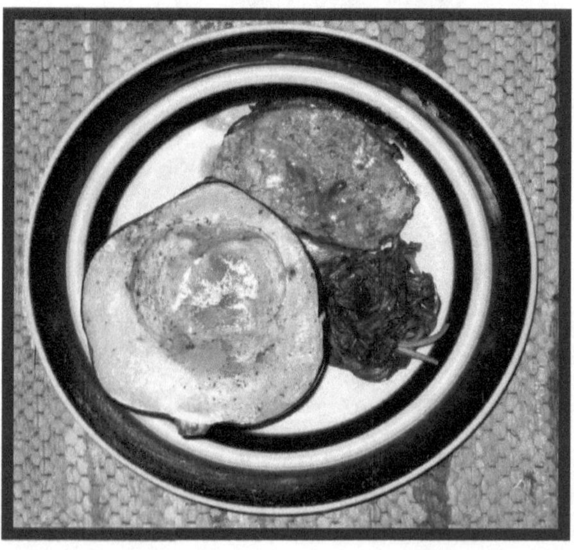

Diet Tip of the Day: **Keep a daily food log** to record everything you eat.
It really does work wonders.

Day 5 Recipe

Frozen-Fish Evening Meal

No recipe today. No cooking today. It's your day off! Some reasonably good frozen fish dinners are:

Shrimp Alfredo	**Lean Cuisine**	~~230~~ 240
Tuna Noodle Casserole	**Smart Ones**	~~250~~ 270
Shrimp & Angel Hair Pasta	**Lean Cuisine**	~~280~~ 290
Parmesan Crusted Fish	**Lean Cuisine**	~~290~~ 300
Tortilla Crusted Fish	**Lean Cuisine**	~~300~~ 310

That's it. At this writing, there are just not that many frozen fish dinners for sale at supermarkets, although new entrees are being introduced continually. If you choose any of the above entrees, you will not use all of the **340 kcal allocated for this meal**. In this case, use the excess calories anyway you wish. Splurge on extra dessert or save the calories for another day! For additional selections see Appendix A on page 104.

If the above frozen entrees are not obtainable in the country where you reside, substitute a locally available frozen dinner with approximately the same calorie count specified in daily menu 5.

Please read the important **Frozen-Food Safety Warning** in Appendix B on page 109.

<u>Diet Tip of the Day:</u> **Buy a pedometer** (or get a pedometer App for your smart phone) and start walking. For the average person 2100 steps amounts to walking about one mile. A Harvard study has shown that 8000 to 10000 step per day promote weight loss. And you're not obliged to walk continuously until you accrue all 10000 steps. Rather, all steps throughout the day to wherever and whenever count toward your daily total. Because 10000 steps a day may not be achievable by some people, particularly those who are elderly, sedentary, or who have chronic diseases, rather than insisting on a blanket 10000 steps per day, your initial stepping goal should your baseline steps plus an increment of an additional 2500 steps. (Your baseline being the number of steps you take in an average day.)

Day 6 Recipe

Grandma's Pizza

The following is a pizza recipe used by my Italian grandmother. She was from a small mountain village located between Rome and Naples.

Pizza dough: To save time use prepared dough, preferably whole grain. Flour a large cutting board. <u>Divide 500 grams of prepared pizza dough into four parts</u>. Roll out each dough ball as thin as possible.

Tomato sauce: Sauté ½ small onion, chopped fine, in 1 tsp (5 mL) olive oil. Add two finely chopped garlic cloves, 200 grams chopped plum tomatoes and small amount of chopped fresh oregano. Stir and cook about 5 minutes on a low flame.

Pizza preparation & cooking: On each pizza, spread evenly about ¼ cup (60 mL) of the tomato sauce. Add about 15 grams of shredded part-skim mozzarella cheese, small amount of Parmesan cheese, 3 slices of a Portobello mushroom, some torn fresh basil, and drizzle with Evoo. Put pizzas on a pan and place in 250 °C oven for about 15 to 20 minutes, or until crust is crisp and cheese is just melting. (Freeze left over sauce for use on Day 13.)

<u>Serves 4</u>. Make four pizzas. Each pizza contains about 350 kcal.

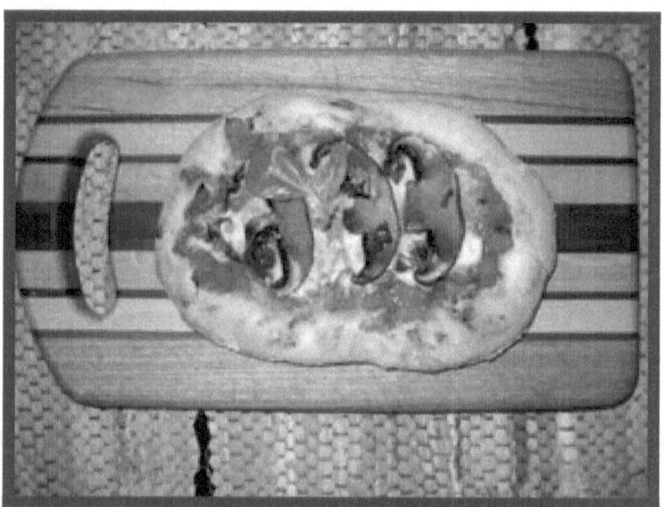

<u>Diet Tip of the Day:</u> For **life-long weight control** take a vigorous 30 to 60 minute walk everyday! That's right – everyday. Make exercise a nonflexible top priority part of your life. When it comes to exercise the key words are consistent, persistent, unyielding, dogged. Get the point?

Day 7 Recipe

Chicken Evening Meal - Out

No recipe today. No cooking today. Have a chicken dinner at your favorite restaurant, but make sure you choose a restaurant where you have a fighting chance to achieve your calorie goal. Your goal for dinner is a **maximum of 630 kcal**. This includes appetizer, soup, main course and dessert.

Tips for Eating Out: First, order simple, such as broiled chicken breast with steamed vegetables and brown rice. Tell the waiter you want no sauce, no gravy, nothing added. Then, knowing your calorie objective, and that chicken is about 200 kcal per 100 grams, most steamed vegetable servings average approximately 40 kcal per 100 grams, and rice is about 120 kcal per 100 grams, decide how much to eat – and take the remainder home. If fresh fruit is not an option, pass on dessert and have the evening snack specified for that day in the diet.

In a restaurant, some nutritionists recommend you eat the low-calorie items on your plate first. Start with the salad, soup and veggies. By the time you get to the chicken and starches you will hopefully be full enough to be content with smaller portions of the higher-calorie choices.

Finally, some dieticians advise their dieting clients not to eat out. That's right. They believe eating at home is safer. But our thought is you have to eat out eventually so why not learn how while your resolve is high?

<u>Diet Tip of the Day:</u> When you're on a diet, eating in a restaurant can be a challenge, because most restaurant portions are huge, and can easily total more than 1000 kcal. When eating in a restaurant decide how much to eat – and take the remainder home. A good general rule of thumb is to **eat half and bring the remainder home**.

Day 8 Recipe

Baked Salmon with Salsa

This is a simple, straight-forward recipe. Again, the advantage of a simple recipe is there are no hidden calories.

4 150 gram salmon fillets

6 Tbsp (90 mL) bottled tomato-pepper salsa

Brown salmon fillets in non-stick pan and place in baking dish. Put fillets in an oven preheated to 175 °C for about 10 minutes. Plate the salmon. Stir prepared tomato-pepper salsa and spoon it over the salmon.

Serves 4. One salmon fillet is about 215 kcal.

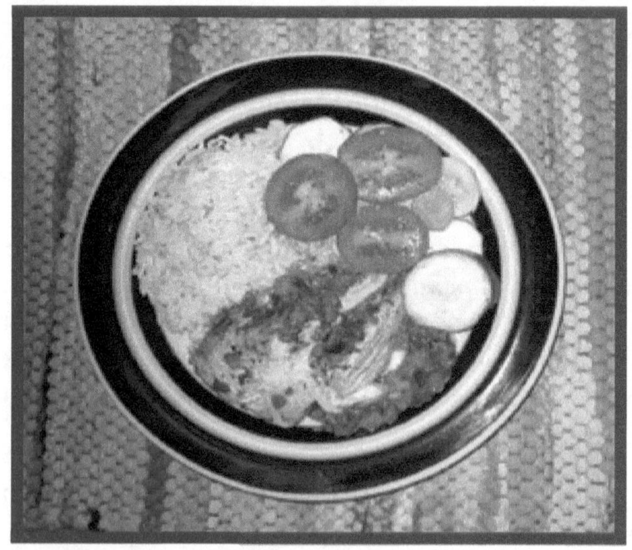

Diet Tip of the Day: **Have soup more often.** Most non-cream-based soups are filling and low-calorie.

Day 9 Recipe

Veggie Burger

Vegetable-based burgers can be purchased at your local supermarket. The patty of a veggie burger can be made from vegetables, soy, nuts, mushrooms, textured vegetable protein, dairy, or a combination of these foods.

Two popular veggie burgers in the U.S. (and Canada) are the Boca Burger and Gardenburger. The Boca Burger is made chiefly from soy protein and grain gluten. (Boca Burger patties range from 60 to 90 kcal.) The original Gardenburger is made from mushrooms, onions, brown rice, rolled oats, cheese, and spices. (Gardenburger patties about 100 kcal.)

Fry's Range burger is popular in the UK. Their original burger is about 100 kcal. Lots of other countries have similar products.

To prepare, follow package directions. The version shown below has an added slice of low-fat cheddar cheese. The lettuce, tomato and ketchup shown actually add very few extra calories.

The veggie burger patty plus low-fat cheese amounts to approximately 150 Calories. Add a seeded roll and the total rises to 290 kcal.

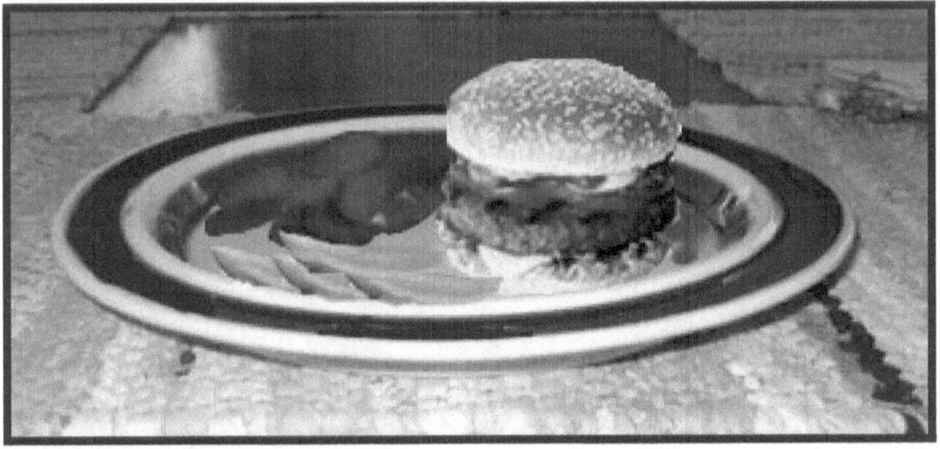

Diet Tip of the Day: **Drink lots of water** – about 8 glasses per day. Add a slice of lemon to make it more interesting. Often, when you think you're hungry, you are just thirsty. So, next time you head for a snack, drink some water first and see if that does it for you.

Day 10 Recipe

Wild Blueberry Pancakes

This recipe makes a relatively low calorie, wholesome batch of delicious wild blueberry-whole grain-buttermilk pancakes.

1 cup (125 grams) whole-grain flour

1 cup (240 mL) buttermilk

1 egg

1 Tbsp (15 mL) vegetable oil

1 tsp (10 grams) baking powder

½ tsp (5 grams) baking soda

Stir ingredients until blended. Add ¾ cup (100 grams) blueberries and gently stir. Using medium heat, preheat a non-stick skillet coated with cooking spray. Pour slightly less than ¼ cup of batter onto skillet per pancake. Cook slowly until bubbles break on surface of pancake. Turn and cook until other side is lightly browned. Makes 8 pancakes. Pictured below are wild-blueberry pancakes with two slices of turkey bacon.

Serves 4. Each pancake is about 95 kcal.

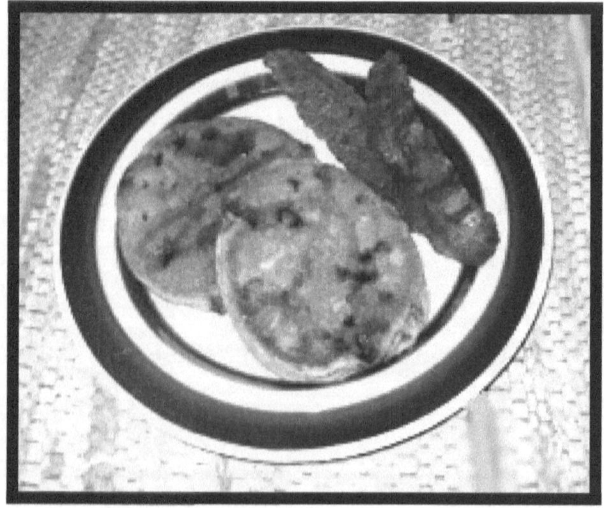

Diet Tip of the Day: A peanut butter sandwich on whole grain bread with a glass of skim milk and an apple makes a nutritious, reasonably low-calorie Mid-Day Meal.

Day 11 Recipe

Artichoke-Bean Salad

500 grams white kidney beans
10 artichoke hearts, quartered
⅓ cup (80 mL) chopped oregano
⅓ cup (80 mL) chopped parsley
3 cloves garlic, chopped
1 lemon, juiced
Combine ingredients in medium-size bowl. Stir in ¼ cup (60 mL) Evoo.
Salt and black pepper to taste.
Serves 6. Artichoke-bean salad has approximately 190 kcal per serving.
Pictured on the plate below are two grilled chicken sausage links with
salsa, steamed green beans and the artichoke-bean salad. Incidentally,
this artichoke-bean combination over mixed salad greens served with a
whole-grain bread makes a delicious, nutritious and reasonable low-
calorie main course.

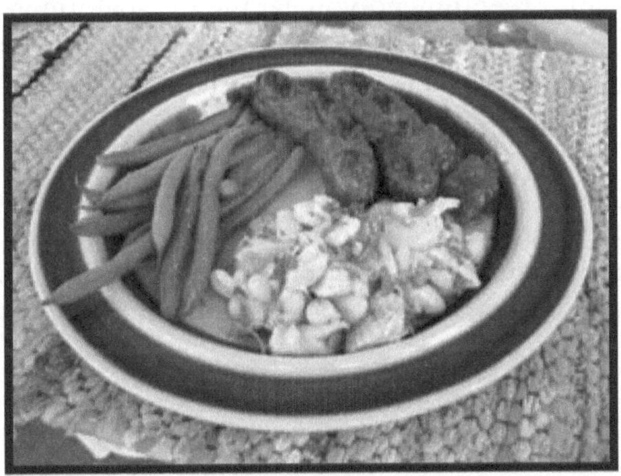

Diet Tip of the Day: Have a small meal before you go to a party. A
hardboiled egg, an apple, and a thirst quencher (like water, tea, seltzer, or
diet soda) will take the edge off your appetite and make it easier to resist
the high-calorie goodies.

Day 12 Recipe
Fish Evening Meal - Out

No recipe today. No cooking today. Have a fish dinner at your favorite
restaurant, but make sure you choose a restaurant where you have a good
chance to achieve your calorie goal. For Day 12, your **goal for dinner is a
maximum of 595 kcal**. This includes appetizer, soup, main course and
dessert.

Tips for Eating Out: The following is almost an exact repeat of advice
given for Day 7. First, order simple, such as broiled fish with steamed
vegetables and brown rice. Tell the waiter you want no sauce, no gravy,
nothing added. Then, knowing your calorie objective, and that most fish is
about 200 kcal per 100 grams, most steamed vegetable servings average
approximately 50 kcal per 100 grams, and rice is about 100 kcal per 100
grams, decide how much to eat – and take the remainder home. If fresh
fruit is not an option, pass on dessert and have the evening snack specified
for that day in the diet.

In a restaurant, I recommend you eat the low-calorie items on your
plate first. Start with the salad, soup and veggies. By the time you get to
the fish and starches you will hopefully be full enough to be content with
smaller portions of the higher-calorie choices.

<u>**Diet Tip of the Day:**</u> Phytonutrients are found in plant foods such as
fruits, vegetables, whole grains, dried beans, nuts and seeds. Unlike
protein, fat, vitamins and minerals, phytonutrients are not necessary for
life, but evidence is growing that phytonutrients have many beneficial
qualities.

Day 13 Recipe

Pasta with Marinara Sauce

Prepare the sauce as you did for the Day 6 pizza (see page 79). But because the pizza sauce is a bit too thick, add 60 mL of pasta liquid to thin it. (The spiral pasta shape shown below is called Fusilli, and is my favorite because all the ridges really hold the sauce.)

½ pound (225 grams) <u>whole-grain</u> pasta

¼ tsp salt

Bring 2 quarts of lightly salted water to a boil. Add pasta and stir occasionally (to keep pasta from sticking to the bottom of the pot). Keep water boiling and cook until pasta are "al dente." (Cooking time is approximately 9 minutes.) Drain pasta, add marinara sauce and serve hot. <u>**Serves 4**</u>. One serving is about 225 kcal.

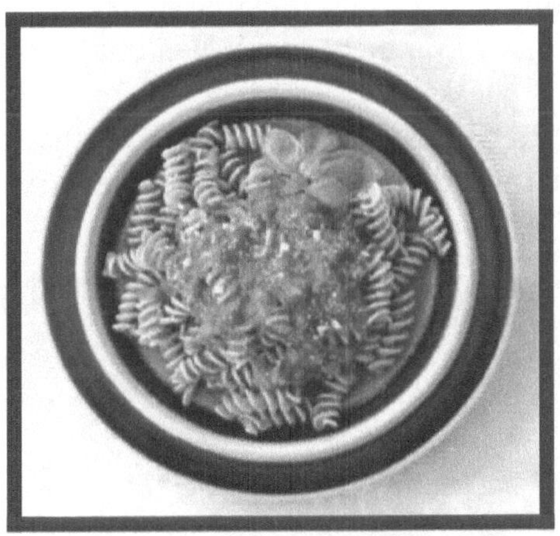

<u>**Diet Tip of the Day:**</u> **Beware of alcoholic beverages**. Beer has about 13 kcal per ounce (30 mL), wine 25 kcal per ounce (30 mL) and whiskey 71 kcal per ounce (30 mL).

Day 14 Recipe

"Oatena" Cereal Mix

Mixing nutritious cereals, hot or cold, is a good way to add variety as well as nutrition to a meal. This recipe features a mix of two whole grain cereals: Oatmeal and Wheatena.

⅓ cup (80 mL) Oatmeal
¼ cup (60 mL) Wheatena
¾ cup (180 mL) water
½ cup (120 mL) skim (fat-free) milk
¼ cup (60 mL) blueberries
10 raisins

Add Oatmeal, Wheatena, raisins and a dash of salt to a microwave-safe cereal bowl. Next add water and stir. Place bowl in microwave, on high power for about 1½ minutes, or until desired consistency is reached. The result is "Oatena," a mix of oatmeal and Wheatena, shown (half eaten) below.

Add skim milk and blueberries and serve hot. Because of the natural sugar in blueberries and raisins, adding sugar is not necessary.

<u>Serves 1</u>. About 310 kcal per serving

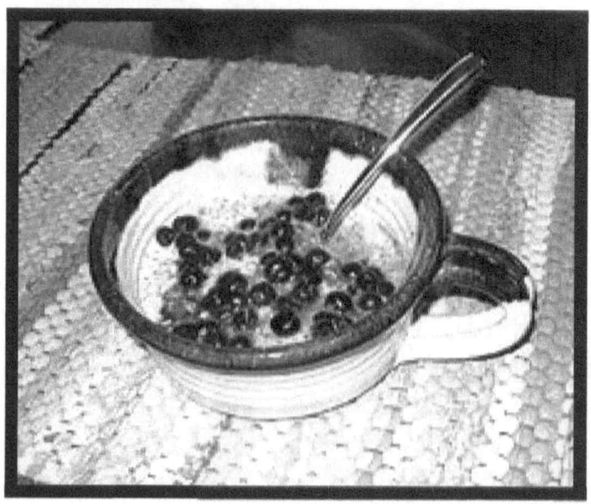

<u>Diet Tip of the Day:</u> Hot or cold cereal topped with fruit, and fat-free milk makes a nutritious, relatively low-calorie meal anytime.

Day 15 Recipe

London Broil

1 pound (450 grams) boneless flank steak about ¾" thick, trimmed of fat
1 clove garlic
1 tsp dry oregano
Rub each side of the flank steak with garlic. Season with oregano, salt
and pepper to taste. Prepare a large non-stick skillet over high heat.
Steak should sizzle when placed on hot skillet. Sear steak on one side for
about 5 minutes; then turn and sear other side for about 4 minutes, or until
done to preference. Check the center by making small incision. Carve
into ¼-inch slices.
Serves 4. About 320 kcal per serving (for meat only).

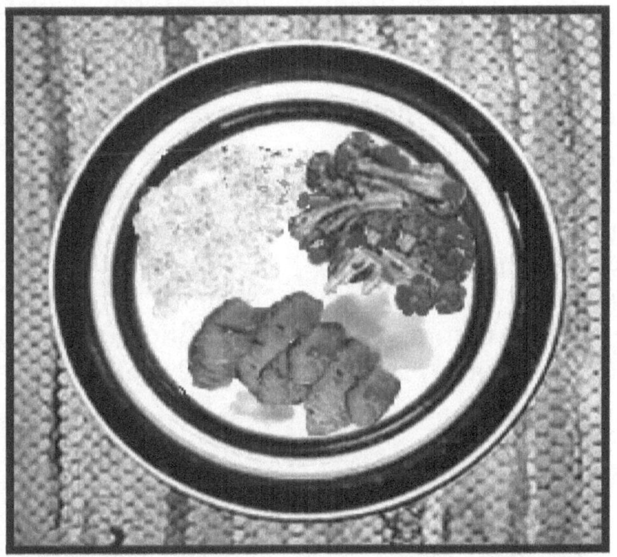

Diet Tip of the Day: Stay Busy. Most people will do anything to avoid
work, housework, yard work, exercise, etc. But any kind of work burns a
lot more calories than just sitting! Whatever it is you are avoiding – just
go do it!

Day 16 Recipe

Baked Red Snapper

4 red snapper fillets – 4 oz (120 grams) each - or salmon fillets.
(salmon may be substituted)
½ cup (120 mL) white wine
½ cup (80 grams) non-fat yogurt mixed with half as much mustard
½ pound (225 grams) green beans
20 cherry tomatoes
4 tsp (20 mL) olive oil
1 cup (200 grams) wild rice, brown rice and grain berry mix
Prepare rice mix per package directions.
Brown fillets in non-stick pan. Place fillets skin side down in baking dish coated with non-stick spray. Add white wine and cook in oven preheated to 175 ºC for about 15 minutes. Spoon pan juices over fillets. Salt and pepper to taste.
Place green beans in skillet. Add ½-cm of water and cook over medium heat until water boils off. Add cherry tomatoes and olive oil. Stir well and sauté for a few minutes. Season with fresh rosemary and oregano. Salt and pepper to taste.
Plate red snapper fillet and spoon over yogurt-mustard sauce. Add green beans & tomato mix and the wild rice. Serve hot.
Serves 4. One plate consisting of one snapper fillet (215 kcal) with green beans & tomato mix (75 kcal) and wild rice (160 kcal) totals 450 kcal.

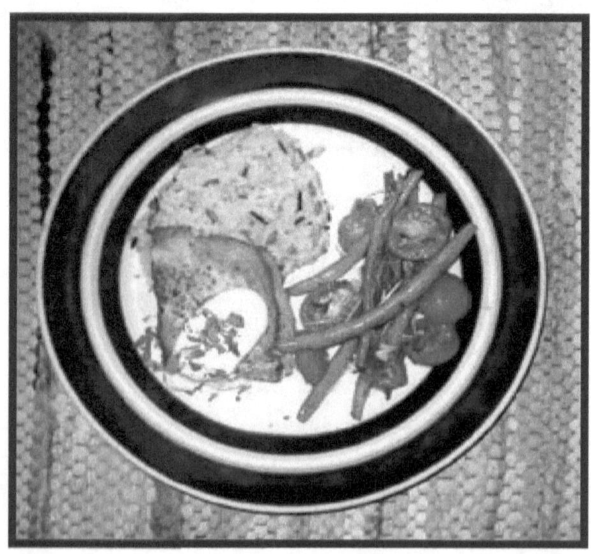

Day 17 Recipe

Cajun Chicken Salad

This is a perfect after-work, quick, nutritious and delicious dinner.

4 boneless and skinless chicken breasts (about 150 grams each)

1 bottle Cajun spices

200 grams mixed salad greens

20 cherry tomatoes

12 pitted black olives

Brush chicken breasts lightly with olive oil. Roll breasts in Cajun spices.
Brown breasts on non-stick oven-proof skillet. After breasts are brown,
put skillet in 175 °C oven for approximately 15 minutes, or until done.
Cut breasts into ½-inch slices. (When the breasts are done, the meat
should be moist and white with no sign of pink.) Serve hot or keep in an
oven or warmer at 100 °C until ready to plate.

Place chicken slices over a bed of mixed salad greens. Add tomatoes,
olives and 2 Tbsp of your favorite low-calorie salad dressing (see page 6).
Serves 4. 330 kcal per serving.

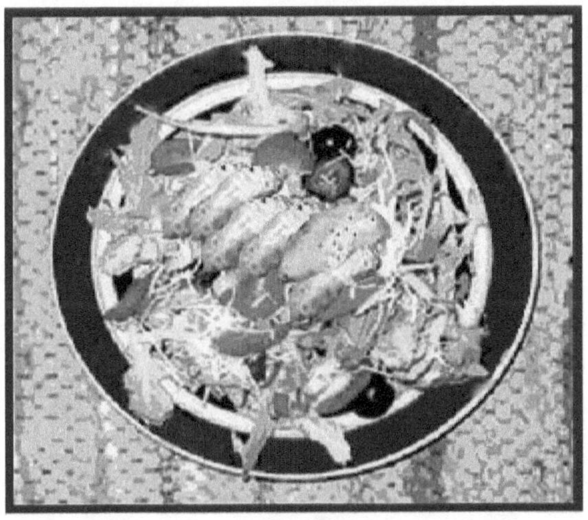

Diet Tip of the Day: Know that **fat-free isn't always your best bet.**
Very often sugar is substituted for fat and the calorie total remains the
same. Low fat does not necessarily mean low calorie! Rather, look for
low-calorie or reduced-calorie products.

Day 18 Recipe

Grilled Swordfish

550 grams swordfish
1 bottle citrus-herb marinade
24 cherry tomatoes
4 medium potatoes
250 grams fresh spinach
1 pinch rosemary & juice of ¼ lemon
10 mL extra virgin olive oil (Evoo)
Steam spinach with garlic and drizzle with Evoo. Cut up potatoes and place sprinkle with lemon juice, add rosemary, salt and black pepper. Place on grill for about 10 minutes, turning occasionally.
Toss cherry tomatoes in small amount Evoo. Add fresh oregano, salt and black pepper. Place on heavy-duty aluminum foil, seal and grill for about 3 minutes.
Marinade swordfish in citrus-herb vinaigrette. Then grill on hot fire for about 5 minutes on one side and 3 minutes on the other, or until done as desired.
Serves 4. One plate consisting of grilled swordfish (250 kcal) with grilled potatoes (100 kcal) and cherry tomatoes (45 kcal) and steamed spinach (50 kcal) totals 445 kcal.

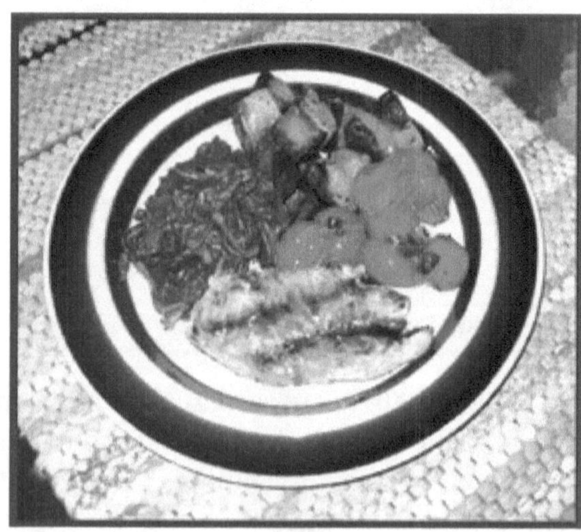

Diet Tip of the Day: Don't be in a hurry to lose weight. Slow weight loss is healthier, is more likely to be permanent, and is easier to sustain over the long haul.

Day 19 Recipe

Chinese Food - Out

No recipe today. No cooking today. Have a Chinese dinner at your favorite restaurant, but make sure you choose a restaurant where you have a reasonable chance to achieve your calorie goal. For today, **your goal for dinner is a maximum of 640 Calories**. This includes any appetizer, soup, main course and any dessert.

Tips for Eating Chinese: You can consume a lot of calories in a Chinese restaurant – if you order carelessly. For example a typical portion of General Tso's chicken is loaded with about 1000 kcal, then add another 200 kcal for a cup of rice.

First rule, order simple. Look for a dish with lots of vegetables, some fish or chicken and brown rice. Tell the waiter you want your food steamed with any sauce on the side. (This is not only a low-calorie way of eating Chinese food but is also the most nutritious way to eat Chinese.)

Then, knowing your 640 kcal objective, and that chicken and fish are about chicken is about 200 kcal per 100 grams, most steamed vegetable servings average approximately 40 kcal per 100 grams, and rice is about 120 kcal per 100 grams, decide how much of the meal you can eat – and take the remainder home. Pass on dessert and have the evening snack specified for that day in the diet. Also see section on **Eating Out on page 8** for more guidance.

<u>Diet Tip of the Day:</u>   Another dilemma for dieters is **judging portion size**. It makes no sense to worry about whether to apportion 70 or 80 kcal per 100 grams for a cut of meat if you have no idea whether the portion you are planning to eat weighs four or ten ounces. To be successful, you must learn to estimate portion sizes with reasonable accuracy.

Day 20 Recipe

Quick Pasta alla Puttanesca

This famous pasta dish originated in Naples. Puttanesca means "ladies of the night." The exact origin of the name is unclear, but one thing is clear: It's delicious! Here is one of many recipe versions.

250 grams spaghetti (whole grain preferred)

20 black pitted olives

1 can (450 grams) diced tomatoes

½ can (120 mL) tomato sauce

30 mL Evoo

3 cloves of garlic, chopped and 1Tbsp dried minced onion

½ tsp crushed red pepper flakes

1 Tbsp capers drained and rinsed

50 grams currants

Cook spaghetti according to package directions. Drain and return spaghetti to pot; add 5 mL Evoo and toss to coat.

Heat 30 mL olive oil in large skillet over medium-high heat. Add red pepper flakes; cook and stir 1 to 2 minutes or until sizzling. Add onion and garlic; cook and stir 1 minute. Finally, add tomatoes with juice, tomato sauce, olives, currants and capers. Cook over medium-high heat, stirring frequently, until sauce is heated through.

Serves 4. About 345 kcal per serving

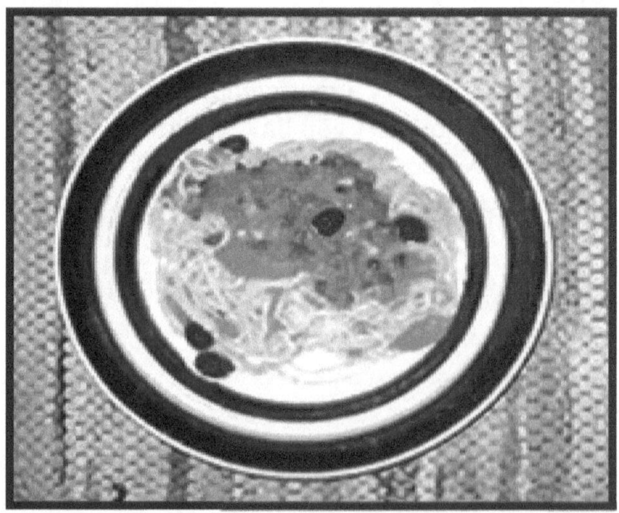

Diet Tip of the Day: Dilute juices, such as apple juice, orange, etc. with water. This cuts the flavor slightly but really reduces calorie content.

Day 21 Recipe

Frozen-Meat Evening Meal

No recipe today. No cooking today. Another day off! That's it. At this writing, there are just not that many frozen meat dinners for sale at supermarkets, although new entrees are being introduced continually. Here are some reasonably good frozen-meat dinners:

Meat	Steak Portobella	Lean Cuisine	160
Meat	Asian Style Beef & Broccoli	Smart Ones	170
Meat	Beef Merlot	Healthy Choice	180
Meat	Homestyle Beef Pot Roast	Smart Ones	180
Meat	Salisbury Steak w Mac & Cheese	Lean Cuisine	290
Pasta	Pasta with Swedish Meatballs	Smart Ones	290
Meat	Classic Meat Loaf	Healthy Choice	300

If you choose most of the above entrees, you will fall well short of the **300 Calories allocated for this day**. In this case, use the remaining calories anyway you wish. Indulge on extra dessert or save the calories for another day.

If the above frozen entrees are not obtainable in the country where you reside, substitute a locally available frozen dinner with approximately the same calorie count specified in daily menu 21.

Please see the important **Frozen-Food Safety Warning** in Appendix B on page 109.

<u>Diet Tip of the Day:</u> A good understanding of nutrition is not only vital for good health but also will help you control your weight over the long term. For example, did you know that foods that are an "excellent source" of a particular nutrient provide 20% or more of the Recommended Daily Value. Whereas, foods that are a "good source" of a nutrient provide between 10 and 20% of the Recommended Daily Value.

Day 22 Recipe

Shrimp & Spinach Salad

900 grams of shrimp in shell
225 grams small green beans, trimmed
225 grams baby spinach leaves
2 Tbsp (30 mL) lemon juice
¼ cup (60 mL) Evoo
2 tsp minced fresh dill
1 Tbsp minced green onion

To make vinaigrette, combine lemon juice, olive oil, dill, salt and pepper to taste and whisk until blended. Stir in minced onion and set aside.

Peel, de-vein and butterfly shrimp. Place shrimp in a bowl and add water to cover. Add 1 teaspoon of salt, and let stand for 10 minutes. Drain, rinse, drain again, and dry. Arrange shrimp in broiling pan without a rack. Brush shrimp with a little vinaigrette and place under preheated broiler, about 3 inches from heat. Broil about 3 to 4 minutes, turning shrimp once, or until both sides turn pink.

Remove shrimp from broiler and add remaining vinaigrette and green beans to the broiling pan. Stir to coat shrimp and beans with vinaigrette. Pour warm vinaigrette over spinach and toss quickly. Plate the spinach and arrange shrimp and green beans on top.

Serves 4. 310 kcal per serving.

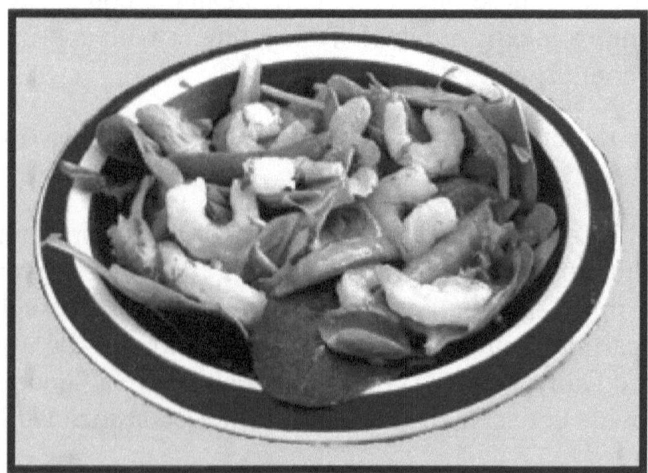

Diet Tip of the Day: When company leaves, have them take some of the leftover food (particularly the dessert) with them – or take the leftovers to work the next day.

Day 23 Recipe

Beans & Greens Salad

⅓ cup chopped oregano
⅓ cup chopped parsley
3 cloves garlic, chopped
1 lemon, juiced
Prepare salad dressing by combining above ingredients and stirring in ¼ cup Evoo. Salt and pepper to taste.
225 grams mesclun mix
110 grams green beans
500 grams canned garbanzo beans (chickpeas)
Arrange mesclun mix, garbanzo beans and green beans on a large platter.
Drizzle salad dressing over beans and greens.
Serves 4. Approximately 260 kcal per serving.

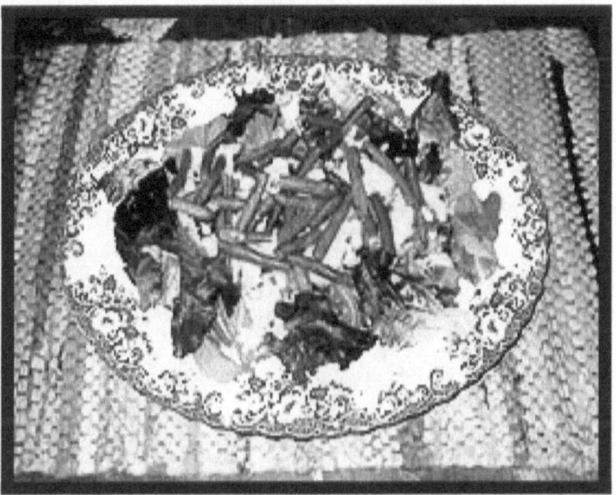

Diet Tip of the Day: Beans are a wonderful food but they are an incomplete protein. If however beans are eaten with a whole-grain bread, the combination forms a complete protein – just as complete and nutritious as meat, poultry, or fish.

Day 24 Recipe

Four-Bean Plus Salad

Note that the total caloric value of the salad will change very little, if the proportions of the bean varieties and corn are varied – according to taste.

½ cup canned red kidney beans, drained and rinsed
½ cup canned black beans, drained and rinsed
½ cup canned chick peas, drained and rinsed
½ cup canned cannelloni beans, drained and rinsed
½ cup canned corn, drained
1 small red pepper, chopped
1 small green pepper, chopped
30 mL Evoo
30 mL lemon juice

In a large bowl mix red kidney beans, black beans, chick peas, cannelloni beans, corn and chopped red and green peppers. Stir in Evoo and lemon juice and plate.

Serves about 6. One serving is 100 grams – with about 135 kcal per serving.

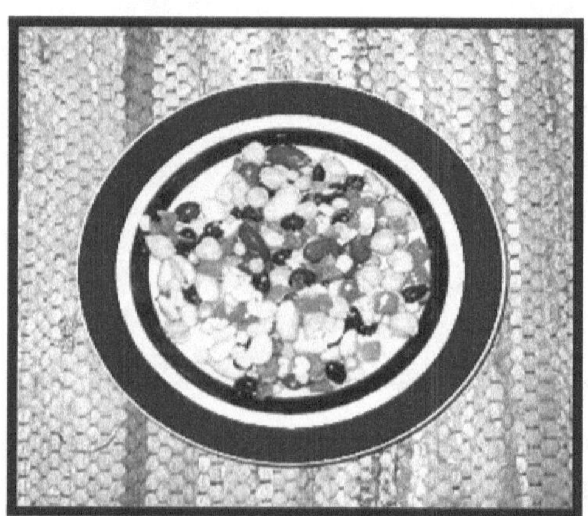

Diet Tip of the Day: Vigorous exercise doesn't necessarily stimulate you to overeat. Just the opposite. In many cases, exercise actually helps curb your appetite – immediately following a workout.

Day 25 Recipe

Pan-Broiled Hanger Steak

600 grams hanger steak, well trimmed of fat
60 mL lime juice
8 small new potatoes, peeled and halved
12 cherry tomatoes, cut in half
Season both sides of steak with salt and pepper and place in sealable
plastic bag with lime juice. Refrigerate for about one hour.

Boil potatoes about 10 minutes. Rinse in cold water. Sauté potatoes in
small amount of vegetable oil over medium-high heat until brown.
Sauté cherry tomatoes in small amount of olive oil over medium-high
heat until skin begins to crack. Season with chopped fresh basil.

Heat a skillet over medium-high heat. Sear hanger steak on one side for
about 5 minutes. Turn over and sear other side approximately 5 minutes
(for medium done). Pour off any fat that may have accumulated. Carve
into ½-inch slices.
Serves 4. About 320 kcal per serving (for the hanger steak only)

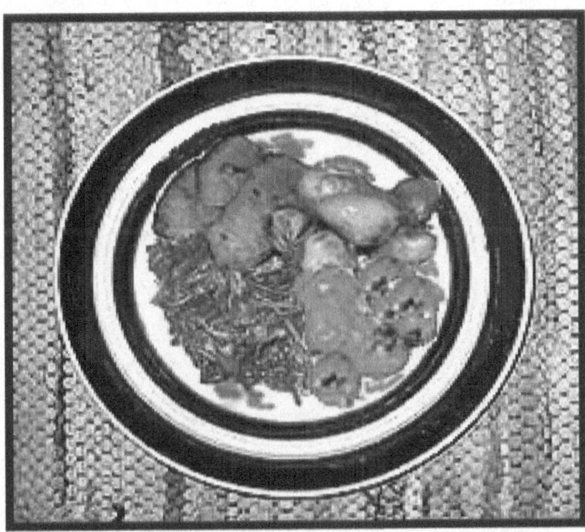

Diet Tip of the Day: If you find yourself at a party, don't stand near the
food! Be aware of the temptation. Make the effort, and you'll find you
eat less.

Day 26 Recipe

Grilled Scallops and Polenta

450 grams of sea scallops
¾ cup polenta cornmeal
180 mL skim milk
1 medium Portobello mushroom
225 grams green beans
40 grams chopped red onion
16 asparagus spears
5 mL Evoo

Bring 360 mL of water and skim milk to rapid boil. Add salt to taste and slowly add polenta while stirring. Reduce heat. Continue stirring until desired consistency is reached. Pour polenta into lightly greased pan. After polenta has cooled cover and refrigerate. Cut chilled polenta into 4 pieces. Grill on medium-hot fire – about two minutes on each side.

Brush Portobello mushroom and asparagus spear with Evoo and place on grill for about 3 minutes on each side.

Grill scallops on medium-hot fire. Turn after two minutes or when first side turns opaque. Grill until second side turns opaque – about another 2 minutes. Don't overcook but test a scallop by cutting to make sure it's cooked through. Salt and pepper to taste.
Serves 4. The food on the plate pictured below totals 380 kcal.

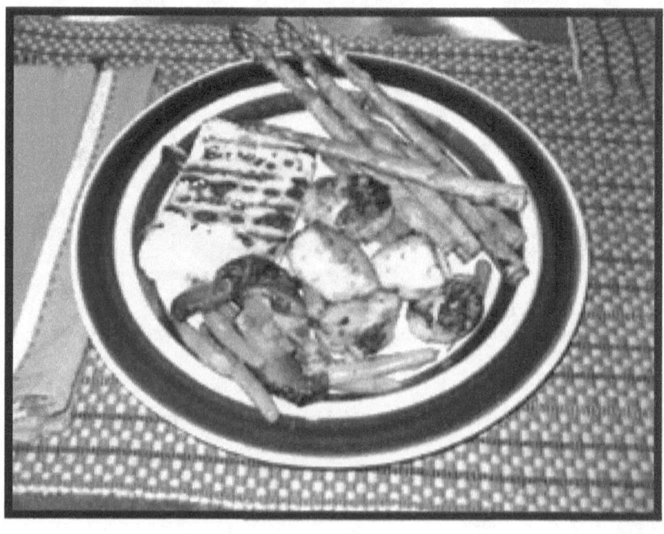

Day 27 Recipe
Fettuccine in Summer Sauce

This sauce is often served in the summer because it's lighter than what is usually dished up with pasta. But despite its name the sauce is wonderful year round.

225 grams fettuccine pasta

225 grams fresh asparagus, trimmed & cut into 5 cm pieces

20 cherry tomatoes, halved

35 mL Evoo

2 cloves of garlic, chopped

½ small onion, diced

Cook fettuccine according to package directions. Drain and return pasta to pot; add 5mL Evoo and toss to coat. Meanwhile steam asparagus and drain.

In large skillet over medium-high heat, sauté cherry tomatoes in 30 mL olive oil until skin begins to crack. Add onion and cook until translucent. Stir in garlic . Thin sauce with pasta liquid to desired consistency. Toss cooked pasta and asparagus into sauce and serve immediately.

Serves 4. About 290 kcal per serving

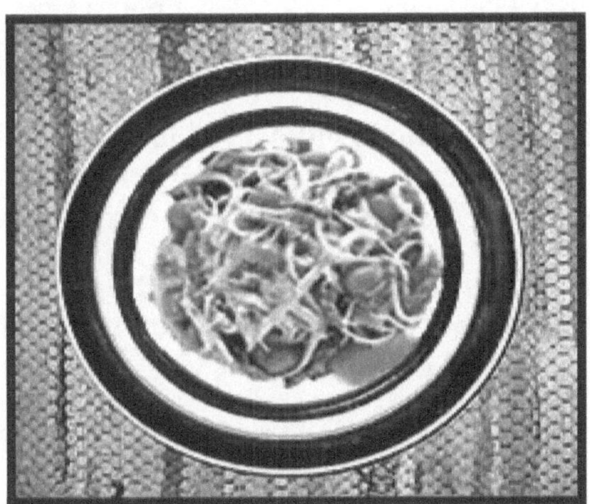

Diet Tip of the Day: A major weight-loss fallacy is that you can get rid of abdominal fat by working your abdominal muscles. This is based on the incorrect belief that fat is eliminated from a particular part of your body if you engage the muscles underneath that layer of fat. No such luck.

Day 28 Recipe

Frozen Chicken Meal

No recipe today. No cooking today. Another day off! There are plenty of frozen chicken choices in your local supermarket. Here are some reasonably good selections:

Poultry	Crustless Chicken Pot Pie	Smart Ones	~~200~~ 190
Poultry	Buffalo Style Chicken	Lean Cuisine	~~200~~ 190
Poultry	Home Style Chicken & Potatoes	Healthy Choice	200
Poultry	Honey Balsamic Chicken	Healthy Choice	210
Poultry	Sesame Stir Fry with Chicken	Lean Cuisine	280
Poultry	Roasted Turkey Breast	Lean Cuisine	~~280~~ 290
Poultry	Apple Cranberry Chicken	Lean Cuisine	280
Poultry	Chicken Fettuccini Alfredo	Healthy Choice	280
Poultry	Grilled Chicken Marinara	Healthy Choice	280
Poultry	Sweet & Spicy Orange Chicken	Healthy Choice	280
Poultry	Chicken Parmesan	Smart Ones	280
Poultry	Turkey Breast with Stuffing	Smart Ones	280

If you fall short of the **300 Calories allocated for today's frozen meal,** use the remaining calories anyway you wish. Overindulge on extra dessert or save the calories for another day.

If the above frozen entrees are not obtainable in the country where you reside, substitute a locally available frozen dinner with approximately the same calorie count specified in daily menu 28.

Please read the important **Frozen-Food Safety Warning** in **Appendix B** on page 109.

<u>Diet Tip of the Day:</u>   The **general weight-change rule is "last on first off."** Assume as you gained weight, the first place you noticed it was on your thighs, next your buttocks, then your face. As you lose weight, it generally will come off in the reverse order, first from your face, then your rear and finally your thighs. And there is not much you can do about that. The truth is there is no food, no exercise, no magic belt, and no pill that will cause your body to lose fat in one place rather than another.

Day 29 Recipe

Barbequed Shrimp

700 grams large shrimp
3 Tbsp bottled barbeque sauce
4 medium ears of corn
Pour barbeque sauce into shallow bowl. Toss shrimp in barbeque sauce to coat. Place shrimp on medium-hot grill. Turn shrimp after about two minutes or when shrimp turn pink. Grill until second side turns pink – approximately another 2 minutes. Don't overcook but test a shrimp by cutting to make sure it is cooked through. Salt and pepper to taste. Serve hot or at room temperature.
Serves 4. About 160 kcal per serving (shrimp only).

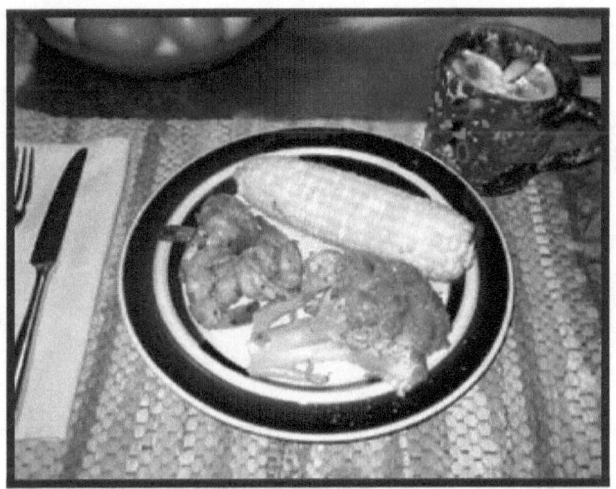

Diet Tip of the Day: A very important weight-profile parameter is your waist-to-hip ratio. Health risks for heart attack and stroke increase considerably for men with a ratio above 1.0 and for women with a ratio above 0.8. To calculate your ratio, measure your waist size (at its narrowest circumference) and divide it by your hip size (at the widest section).

Day 30 Recipe

Cheeseburger

There's really not much to grilling hamburgers. The ideal meat for a juicy burger is ground chuck with about 20% fat, but we are talking diet here. So we opt for leaner, much leaner meat.

600 grams ground sirloin (95% lean)

4 thin slices low-fat cheese

Mix ground beef in large bowl. Salt and pepper to taste. Divide into 4 equal portions and form burgers about 1-inch thick. Cook burgers over a hot fire on charcoal or gas-fired grill. For medium, cook about 4 minutes on each side. Top with slice of cheese.

Serves 4. About 320 kcal per serving (hamburger meat only).

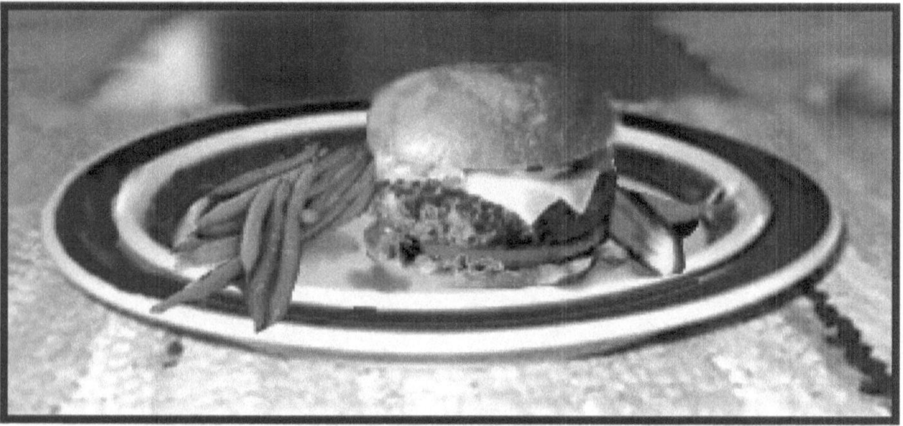

Diet Tip of the Day: Plan to be on a diet the rest of your life. Not necessarily a weight reducing diet. At some point you'll want to just maintain your weight. But you will still need to continue to make good healthy food choices – and not slip back to your old eating habits.

Appendix A: Frozen Entrees

Appendix D lists three popular brands of frozen entrées: Healthy Choice, Lean Cuisine and Smart Ones (Weight Watchers). Note that each brand is color coded. The listing is further divided by entrée type: Poultry entrées, Meat entrées, Seafood entrées, Pasta entrées, Pizza and Other entrées. The entire table is arranged from the lowest to highest in calories. Note that the listed frozen entrées were available in most American and Canadian super markets as of 02/14/2020.

Entrée Type	Name	Brand	Calories
Poultry	Tomato Basil Chicken & Spinach	Smart Ones	160
Meat	Steak Portobella	Lean Cuisine	160
Meat	Asian Style Beef & Broccoli	Smart Ones	~~160~~ 170
Poultry	Herb Roasted Chicken	Lean Cuisine	170
Poultry	Slow Roasted Turkey Breast	Smart Ones	170
Poultry	Grilled Chicken Marsala	Healthy Choice	180
Poultry	Creamy Basil Chicken w Broccoli	Smart Ones	~~180~~ 170
Poultry	Garlic Chicken Rolls	Lean Cuisine	180
Meat	Beef Merlot	Healthy Choice	180
Meat	Homestyle Beef Pot Roast	Smart Ones	180
Poultry	Roasted Turkey & Vegetables	Lean Cuisine	190
Poultry	Chicken & Broccoli Alfredo	Healthy Choice	190
Poultry	Chicken & Vegetable Stir Fry	Healthy Choice	190
Other	Broccoli & Cheddar Roast Potato	Smart Ones	190
Poultry	Home Style Chicken & Potatoes	Healthy Choice	200
Poultry	Crustless Chicken Pot Pie	Smart Ones	~~200~~ 190
Poultry	Buffalo Style Chicken	Lean Cuisine	~~200~~ 190
Pasta	Angel Hair Marinara	Smart Ones	200
Poultry	Salisbury Steak	Smart Ones	200
Meat	Roast Beef & Mashed Potatoes	Smart Ones	~~220~~ 200
Pasta	Primavera Pasta	Smart Ones	210
Poultry	Honey Balsamic Chicken	Healthy Choice	210

Pasta	Ravioli Florentine	Smart Ones	210
Poultry	Cajun Style Chicken & Shrimp	Healthy Choice	220
Pasta	Cheese Ravioli Mushroom Sauce	Smart Ones	230
Poultry	Ranchero Chicken Wrap	Smart Ones	230
Poultry	Lemon Herb Chicken Picante	Smart Ones	230
Pasta	Cheese Ravioli Mushroom Sauce	Smart Ones	230
Meat	Meat Loaf with Mashed Potatoes	Lean Cuisine	~~230~~ 240
Seafood	Shrimp Alfredo	Lean Cuisine	~~230~~ 240
Poultry	Chicken Margherita	Smart Ones	~~220~~ 240
Poultry	Grilled Chicken Caesar	Lean Cuisine	240
Poultry	Honey Glazed Turkey & Potatoes	Healthy Choice	240
Pasta	Spicy Penne Arrabbiata	Lean Cuisine	240
Pasta	Four Cheese Cannelloni	Lean Cuisine	~~240~~ 250
Poultry	Creamy Basil Chicken w Tortellini	Lean Cuisine	~~240~~ 250
Pasta	Cheese Ravioli	Lean Cuisine	250
Pasta	Vermont Cheddar Mac & Cheese	Lean Cuisine	250
Pasta	Fettuccini Alfredo	Smart Ones	250
Poultry	Oriental Chicken	Smart Ones	250
Poultry	Fiesta Grilled Chicken	Lean Cuisine	250
Pasta	Chicken Linguini Red Pepper	Healthy Choice	250
Poultry	Golden Roasted Turkey Breast	Healthy Choice	250
Poultry	Chicken Mesquite	Smart Ones	250
Poultry	Chicken Oriental	Smart Ones	250
Poultry	Orange Sesame Chicken	Smart Ones	250
Poultry	Baked Chicken	Lean Cuisine	~~250~~ 260
Poultry	Teriyaki Chicken & Vegetables	Smart Ones	~~250~~ 260
Seafood	Tuna Noodle Casserole	Smart Ones	~~250~~ 270
Pasta	Spaghetti with Meatballs	Lean Cuisine	260
Poultry	Creamy Chicken & Noodles	Healthy Choice	260
Meat	Barbecue Steak w Red Potatoes	Healthy Choice	260

Pasta	Tortellini Primavera Parmesan	Healthy Choice	260
Pasta	Sesame Noodles with Vegetables	Smart Ones	~~260~~ 280
Pasta	Creamy Rigatoni w Chicken	Smart Ones	260
Pasta	Macaroni & Cheese	Smart Ones	260
Pasta	Butternut Squash Ravioli	Lean Cuisine	260
Other	Santa Fe Rice & Beans	Smart Ones	260
Other	Coconut Chickpea Curry	Lean Cuisine	260
Poultry	Glazed Turkey Tenderloins	Lean Cuisine	270
Poultry	Kung Pao Chicken	Healthy Choice	270
Poultry	Chicken Margherita w Balsamic	Healthy Choice	270
Poultry	Chicken Strips & Sweet Potatoes	Smart Ones	270
Pasta	Spaghetti with Meat Sauce	Smart Ones	~~270~~ 280
Meat	Salisbury Steak with Mac & Cheese	Lean Cuisine	~~270~~ 290
Pasta	Penne Rosa	Lean Cuisine	270
Poultry	Turkey Breast & Stuffing	Smart Ones	~~270~~ 280
Pasta	Classic Macaroni & Beef	Lean Cuisine	270
Pasta	Mushroom Mezzaluna Ravioli	Lean Cuisine	270
Pasta	Pasta with Swedish Meatballs	Smart Ones	~~280~~ 290
Other	Asian Pot Stickers	Lean Cuisine	280
Poultry	Sesame Stir Fry with Chicken	Lean Cuisine	280
Poultry	Roasted Turkey Breast	Lean Cuisine	~~280~~ 290
Poultry	Apple Cranberry Chicken	Lean Cuisine	280
Poultry	Chicken Fettuccini Alfredo	Healthy Choice	280
Poultry	Grilled Chicken Marinara	Healthy Choice	280
Poultry	Sweet & Spicy Orange Chicken	Healthy Choice	280
Poultry	Chicken Parmesan	Smart Ones	280
Poultry	Turkey Breast with Stuffing	Smart Ones	280
Meat	Beef & Broccoli	Healthy Choice	280
Meat	Meatball Marinara	Healthy Choice	280
Meat	Beef Teriyaki	Healthy Choice	280

Pasta	Spinach Artichoke Ravioli	Lean Cuisine	280
Other	Vegetable Fried Rice	Smart Ones	280
Pasta	Spinach Artichoke Ravioli	Lean Cuisine	280
Pasta	Linguini with Ricotta & Spinach	Lean Cuisine	280
Poultry	Chicken Fettuccini	Lean Cuisine	~~290~~ 280
Pasta	Spaghetti & Meatballs	Healthy Choice	280
Pasta	Spaghetti with Meat Sauce	Smart Ones	280
Other	Vegetable Fried Rice	Smart Ones	280
Other	Asian Pot Stickers	Lean Cuisine	280
Poultry	Chicken with Almonds	Lean Cuisine	290
Poultry	Chicken with Peanut Sauce	Lean Cuisine	290
Seafood	Shrimp & Angel Hair Pasta	Lean Cuisine	~~280~~ 290
Poultry	Grilled Chicken Pesto w Veggies	Healthy Choice	290
Poultry	General Tso's Spicy Chicken	Healthy Choice	290
Poultry	Pineapple Chicken	Healthy Choice	290
Poultry	Chicken Enchiladas Suiza	Smart Ones	290
Meat	Swedish Meatballs	Lean Cuisine	290
Seafood	Lemon Pepper Fish	Healthy Choice	290
Pasta	Pasta with Swedish Meatballs	Smart Ones	290
Other	Santa Fe Rice & Beans	Smart Ones	290
Pizza	Thin Crust Cheese Pizza	Smart Ones	290
Seafood	Parmesan Crusted Fish	Lean Cuisine	~~290~~ 300
Pasta	Santa Fe-Style Rice & Beans	Lean Cuisine	~~280~~ 300
Poultry	Roasted Turkey & Vegetables	Lean Cuisine	~~290~~ 300
Poultry	Sweet & Sour Chicken	Lean Cuisine	300
Poultry	Crustless Chicken Pot Pie	Healthy Choice	300
Poultry	Sweet Sesame Chicken	Healthy Choice	300
Poultry	Chicken Fettuccini	Smart Ones	300
Poultry	General Tso's Chicken	Smart Ones	300
Meat	Classic Meat Loaf	Healthy Choice	300
Seafood	Tortilla Crusted Fish	Lean Cuisine	~~300~~ 310

Category	Item	Brand	Calories
Pasta	Tuscan-Style Vegetable Lasagna	Lean Cuisine	~~300~~ 310
Pasta	Tortellini with Red Pepper Sauce	Lean Cuisine	300
Pasta	Broccoli Cheddar Rotini	Lean Cuisine	300
Pasta	Three Cheese Ziti Marinara	Smart Ones	300
Pasta	Lasagna Florentine	Smart Ones	~~310~~ 300
Seafood	Tortilla Crusted Fish	Lean Cuisine	~~300~~ 310
Pasta	Tuscan-Style Vegetable Lasagna	Lean Cuisine	~~300~~ 310
Poultry	Chicken Fried Rice	Lean Cuisine	~~300~~ 310
Poultry	Orange Chicken	Lean Cuisine	310
Poultry	Chicken Tikka Masala	Lean Cuisine	310
Poultry	Chicken Strips & Fries	Smart Ones	310
Poultry	Chicken Teriyaki	Lean Cuisine	310
Pizza	Thin Crust Pepperoni Pizza	Smart Ones	310
Pasta	Three Cheese Macaroni	Smart Ones	310
Pizza	French Bread Pepperoni Pizza	Lean Cuisine	310
Poultry	Chicken Spinach Mushroom Panini	Lean Cuisine	~~350~~ 310
Other	Spicy Beef & Bean Enchilada	Lean Cuisine	310
Poultry	Chicken Fried Rice	Healthy Choice	320
Meat	Sweet & Spicy Korean Beef	Lean Cuisine	320
Pizza	Farmers Market Pizza	Lean Cuisine	320
Pizza	Margherita Pizza	Lean Cuisine	320
Poultry	Chicken Carbonara	Lean Cuisine	330
Poultry	Mango Chicken w Coconut Rice	Lean Cuisine	330
Poultry	Country Fried Chicken	Healthy Choice	330
Other	Cheese & Fire-Roasted Tamale	Lean Cuisine	330
Poultry	Chicken Club Panini	Lean Cuisine	~~350~~ 340
Meat	Philly Style Steak & Cheese Panini	Lean Cuisine	~~330~~ 350
Poultry	Chicken Parmigiana	Healthy Choice	360
Poultry	Chicken Pecan	Lean Cuisine	~~320~~ 370
Poultry	Sweet & Sour Chicken	Healthy Choice	390
Pizza	Supreme Pizza	Lean Cuisine	~~330~~ 390

APPENDIX B
Frozen Food Safety

Increasingly, food giants like ConAgra, Nestlé and others that supply consumers with processed foods concede that they cannot ensure the safety of their food products. Frozen foods pose a particularly serious safety problem because unsuspecting consumers buy frozen foods for their convenience and incorrectly believe that cooking frozen foods is a matter of taste – not safety.

Still the food industry says that extensive outbreaks of food-borne illness are rare, even though it is well-known that most of the millions of cases of food-borne illness every year go unreported or are not traced to the source. For example, each year approximately 40,000 cases of salmonella poisoning are reported in the United States – but perhaps as many as one million cases go unreported. (Salmonella is a type of bacteria most often found in poultry, eggs, unprocessed milk, meat and water.) Recently salmonella pathogens in some frozen meals have sickened thousands of people.

How could this happen? First, the supply chain for ingredients in processed foods – from flour to fruits and vegetables to flavorings – is becoming more complex and global in the drive to keep food costs down. As a result, government and industry officials concede that almost every food ingredient is now a potential carrier of pathogens. A further complication is that a large number of food companies subcontract processing work to save money and don't require suppliers to test for pathogens. In fact, companies often don't even know who is supplying their ingredients.

In addition, many frozen-food manufacturers have stopped cooking their products at high temperatures, a tactic they call the "kill step," which is intended to eliminate any lingering microbes. Frequently this process step turns some of the frozen food ingredients into mush. So, instead the "kill step" has been shifted to consumers. For example, ConAgra has added food safety instructions to its frozen meals, including the Healthy Choice brand. A typical "frozen-food safety" instruction offers this guidance: "Internal temperature needs to reach 165°F as measured by a food thermometer in several spots."
Moreover, General Mills, now advises consumers to avoid microwaves altogether and cook their frozen pizzas only in a conventional oven.

Bottom line: To be safe, always cook frozen foods so that the internal temperature reaches 165°F as measured by a good food thermometer.

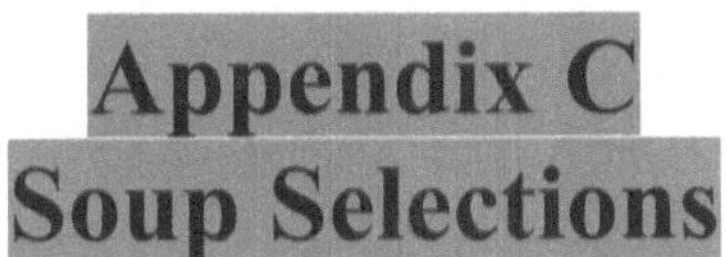

Appendix C
Soup Selections

When the Daily Meal Plan menu specifies soup have only one serving (240 mL) unless stated otherwise. Note that the listed soups were available in most supermarkets as of 02/14/2020.   *These are a canned soup selections.

Soup Description	Calories
Healthy Choice Chicken with Rice	90
Campbell's Tomato	100
Progresso Minestrone*	110
Progresso Chickarina*	110
Progresso Italian-Style Wedding*	120
Campbell's Home-Style Light Chicken Corn Chowder*	120
Campbell's Home-Style Chicken Noodle	130
Campbell's Home-Style Butter Nut Squash*	130
Campbell's Healthy Request Vegetable Beef	140
Progresso Lentil*	140
Progresso Green Split Pea*	150
Campbell's Slow Kettle New England Clam Chowder	160
Progresso Macaroni and Bean*	160
Progresso New England Clam Chowder*	170
Progresso Lasagna-Style*	170
Progresso Broccoli Cheese with Bacon*	180
As an alternative, substitute 2 servings of a 90 Calorie soup	180
Campbell's Chunky Classic Chicken Noodle	190
Amy's Rustic Italian Vegetable*	190
Campbell's Chunky Beef n Cheese*	200
Amy's French Country Vegetable*	210
Campbell's Chunky Sirloin Burger + Vegetables	220
Enjoy two servings of a 110 or 120 Calorie soup	230
Enjoy two servings of a 120 Calorie soup	240

<u>NoPaperPress Paperbacks and eBooks</u>

100-Day Super Diet-1200 Calorie*	Weight Loss for Men - Metric*
100-Day Super Diet-1500 Calorie*	Maximum Weight Loss- 1200 Calorie*
100-Day No-Cooking Diet-1200 Cal*	Maximum Weight Loss- 1500 Calorie*
100-Day No-Cooking Diet-1500 Cal*	Weight Control - U.S. Edition
90-Day Smart Diet-1200 Calorie*	Weight Control - Metric. Edition
90-Day Smart Diet-1500 Calorie*	Professional Weight Control Women - U.S.
90-Day No-Cooking Diet - 1200 Cal*	Professional Weight Control Women - Metric
90-Day No-Cooking Diet - 1500 Cal*	Professional Weight Control Men - U.S.
90-Day Perfect Diet - 1200 Calorie*	Professional Weight Control Men - Metric
90-Day Perfect Diet - 1500 Calorie*	Weight Maintenance - U.S. Edition*
60-Day Perfect Diet-1200 Calorie*	Weight Maintenance - Metric. Edition*
60-Day Perfect Diet-1500 Calorie*	Weight Maintenance - UK Edition
50-Day Flex Diet-1200 Calorie*	Weight Loss for Senior Men*
50-Day Flex Diet-1500 Calorie*	Weight Loss for Senior Women*
30-Day Quick Diet - for Women*	Eat Smart - U.S. Edition*
30-Day Quick Diet - for Men*	Eat Smart - Metric Edition
30-Day No-Cooking Diet*	Eat Smart - UK Edition
30-Day Diet for Women - Metric Ed	Exercise Smart - U.S. Edition
30-Day Diet for Men - Metric Ed	Exercise Smart - Metric Edition
25 Day Easy Diet-1200 Calorie*	Exercise Smart - UK Edition
25 Day Easy Diet-1500 Calorie*	Total Fitness - U.S. Edition
25-Day No-Cooking Diet	Total Fitness - Metric Edition
10-Day Express Diet	Total Fitness - UK Edition
10-Day No-Cooking Diet*	Total Fitness for Women-U.S. Edition*
7-Day Diet for Women*	Total Fitness for Women - Metric
7-Day Diet for Men*	Total Fitness for Women - UK Edition
7-Day No-Cooking Diets*	Total Fitness for Men - U.S. Edition*
90-Day Gluten-Free Diet-1200 Cal*	Total Fitness for Men- Metric Edition*
90-Day Gluten-Free Diet-1500 Cal*	Total Fitness for Men - UK Edition
30-Day Gluten-Free Quick Diet*	Senior Fitness - U.S. Edition*
30-Day Gluten-Free No-Cooking Diet*	Senior Fitness - Metric Edition*
7-Day Diet for Women - Metric	Senior Fitness - UK Edition*
7-Day Diet for Men - Metric	Computer Diet - U.S. Edition*
7-Day Gluten-Free Express Diet*	Computer Diet - Metric Edition*
7-Day Gluten-Free No-Cooking Diet*	Reliable Weight Loss - U.S. Edition
90-Day Vegetarian Diet-1200 Calorie*	Reliable Weight Loss - Metric Edition
90-Day Vegetarian Diet-1500 Calorie*	101 Weight Loss Tips*
30-Day Vegetarian Diet*	101 Healthy Eating Tips*
7-Day Vegetarian Diet*	101 Lifelong Fitness Tips*
Weight Loss for Women*	101 Weight Maintenance Tips
Weight Loss for Women - Metric	101 Weight Loss Recipes
Weight Loss for Women - UK	101 Gluten-Free Weight Loss Recipes
Weight Loss for Men*	101 Vegetarian Weight Loss Recipes*

* These titles are available as both ebooks and paperbacks.

NoPaperPress ebooks sold by Amazon, Apple, Google, Barnes & Noble and Kobo.
NoPaperPress paperbacks are only sold by Amazon.

111

Disclaimer

This book offers general meal planning, nutrition and weight control information. It is not a medical manual and the author does not claim to be medically qualified. The material in this book is not intended to be a substitute for medical counseling. Everyone should have a medical checkup before beginning a weight loss program. Moreover, the physician conducting the medical exam should be made aware of and should approve the specific weight control program planned. Additionally, while the author and publisher have made every effort to ensure the accuracy of the information in this book, they make no representations or warranties regarding its accuracy or completeness. Further, neither the author nor publisher assume liability for any medical problems that might result from applying the methods in this book, or for any loss of profit, or any other commercial damages, including but not limited to special, incidental, consequential or other damages, and any such liability is hereby expressly disclaimed.